Ageing, Physical Activity and Health

T0188256

One of the most pressing questions facing society today is how to care for its burgeoning elderly population. By the year 2050, experts predict that one-third of the world's population will be over 60 years old. Health promotion for the elderly is therefore becoming an increasingly important topic in public policy and planning.

This book examines the challenges presented by an ageing global population, our varying expectations of healthy ageing, and the importance of exercise and physical activity for the elderly. Drawing on empirical research from around the world, it considers the factors that influence health and well-being in later life and compares practices and policies designed to promote healthy ageing. It presents case studies from 15 countries spanning Europe, North and South America, Africa and Asia, and sheds light on how attitudes to physical activity differ across nations, regions and cultures.

Ageing, Physical Activity and Health: International Perspectives is important reading for all students, researchers and practitioners with an interest in physical activity, public health, exercise science or gerontology.

Karin Volkwein-Caplan is Professor in the Department of Kinesiology at West Chester University of Pennsylvania, USA. She has published extensively on gender, HIV/AIDS and Sport, Sexual Harassment in Sport, Ethics in Sport, as well as Healthy Aging and Fitness. Her publications include more than 60 articles as well as 10 book volumes. She is also co-editor of two book series: "Sport, Culture and Society" and "Healthy Aging and Fitness" and has served on the Editorial Board of the International Council of Sport Science and Physical Education since 2012.

Jasmin Tahmaseb McConatha is Professor in the Department of Psychology at West Chester University of Pennsylvania, USA. She specializes in adult development, gerontology and cultural psychology. For 25 years she has conducted research and taught courses on culture, ageing and well-being. This work has resulted in dozens of published papers, chapters and three books. She directs a World Health sponsored "Age Friendly Communities" project in West Chester, Pennsylvania. Dr. Tahmaseb McConatha is an advocate for the rights of older men and women from diverse backgrounds in their fight against ageist practices and policies. She is co-editor of two books series: "Healthy Aging and Fitness" and "Sport, Culture and Society."

ICSSPE Perspectives

The Multidisciplinary Series of Physical Education and Sport Science

The ICSSPE Perspectives series aims to facilitate the application of sport scientific findings to practical areas of sport by integrating a wide variety of fields. Each volume in the series contains expert contributions from different disciplines and different countries addressing a specific topic. The themes of the series come from members, partners, and friends of the ICSSPE and are evaluated by its Development Committee.

Also available in this series:

Published by ICSSPE – www.icsspe.org

Sport for Persons with a Disability
Edited by Colin Higgs and Yves Vanlandewijck

Talent Identification and Development
The Search for Sporting Excellence
Edited by Richard Fisher and Richard Bailey

Published by Routledge – www.routledge.com/sport

Sport and Health
Exploring the Current State of Play
Edited by Daniel Parnell and Peter Krustrup

Ageing, Physical Activity and Health
International Perspectives
Edited by Karin Volkwein-Caplan and Jasmin Tahmaseb McConatha

www.routledge.com/sport/series/ICSSPE

Ageing, Physical Activity and Health

International Perspectives

Edited by
Karin Volkwein-Caplan and
Jasmin Tahmaseb McConatha

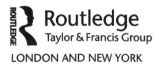
Routledge
Taylor & Francis Group
LONDON AND NEW YORK

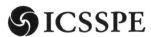 ICSSPE

First published 2018 by Routledge

2 Park Square, Milton Park, Abingdon, Oxfordshire OX14 4RN

52 Vanderbilt Avenue, New York, NY 10017

Routledge is an imprint of the Taylor & Francis Group, an informa business

First issued in paperback 2019

British Library Cataloguing-in-Publication Data
A catalogue record for this book is available from the British Library

Library of Congress Cataloging-in-Publication Data
Names: Volkwein-Caplan, Karin A. E., editor.
Title: Ageing, physical activity and health : international perspectives / edited by Karin Volkwein-Caplan and Jasmin Tahmaseb McConatha.
Description: Milton Park, Abingdon, Oxon ; New York, NY : Routledge, 2018. |
Series: ICSSPE perspectives | Includes bibliographical references and index.
Identifiers: LCCN 2017050769| ISBN 9781138052130 (hbk) | ISBN 9781315167992 (ebk)
Subjects: LCSH: Aging–Health aspects. | Older people–Health and hygiene. | Exercise for older people.
Classification: LCC RA564.8 .A425 2018 | DDC 613.7/10846–dc23
LC record available at https://lccn.loc.gov/2017050769

ISBN: 978-1-138-05213-0 (hbk)
ISBN: 978-0-367-89416-0 (pbk)

Typeset in Sabon
by Wearset Ltd, Boldon, Tyne and Wear

We would like to dedicate this work to our parents and role models for staying physically active at any age: Margarete and Hans-Heinrich Volkwein, and Ulla and Aziz Bani Tahmasab

Contents

**Chronic conditions and the impact of physical
activity and exercise**   161

12 Coping with chronic illness in the twenty-first century:
    the global diabetes crisis   163
    JASMIN TAHMASEB McCONATHA AND
    ELIZABETH RAYMOND

13 Education, physical activity, and healthy aging in Italy:
    theoretical and operating dimensions   175
    ANTONIA CUNTI AND SERGIO BELLANTONIO

14 Achieving active and healthy aging in Sri Lanka   189
    MALATHIE P. DISSANAYAKE

    Conclusion   205
    KARIN VOLKWEIN-CAPLAN AND
    JASMIN TAHMASEB McCONATHA

    Index   209

Contributors

Amarachi Akwarandu is a graduate student with a focus on clinical psychology in the Department of Psychology at West Chester University of Pennsylvania. She holds a Bachelor's in Psychology from Rutgers University, 2015. She works under the guidance of Dr. Tahmaseb McConatha as the project coordinator for ILEARN, an intergenerational learning project sponsored by the World Health Organization and American Association of Retired People (AARP), connecting generations and communities. Her research interests include immigration and acculturation effect on children and families.

Anabela Almeida holds a PhD in Management from the University of Beira Interior, Covilhã/Portugal. From 2012 to 2015 she was a member of the executive board of Cova da Beira Hospital Center–Academic hospital. She is a researcher at the research center of University of Beira Interior (NECE–UBI), participating in several research projects with different research groups and institutions. Her research interests include evaluation of health performance; measurement of health results; quality of life and health indicators. She has participated in many conferences and published several papers in peer-review journals.

Richmond Aryeetey is Senior Lecturer with the University of Ghana School of Public Health. He is trained as a public health nutritionist with an interest in nutritional epidemiology and community nutrition. Areas of research interest include malnutrition across the lifecycle, nutrition and food security, physical activity and ecological determinants of malnutrition focusing on policy and institutional strengthening to address malnutrition. He is currently active in promoting the use of evidence for decisions in nutrition and health in Africa through his work with the EVIDENT collaboration.

Delali Margaret Badasu is Director of the Centre for Migration Studies at the University of Ghana and Senior Research Fellow at the Regional Institute for Population Studies at the same university. She holds a

PhD in Geography and Resource Development from the University of Ghana where she earlier obtained her Bachelor's (Hons) Economics/ Geography and Master's (Population Studies). She also holds a Master's (Geography) from the University of Alberta, Canada and Post Graduate Diploma in Social Policy from the Institute for Social Studies (ISS), The Hague. Her research interest covers various issues in family studies such as care for children and the health and nutritional outcomes and well-being of mothers of migrant families. Her major areas of research interest in migration include migration and development; migration and the family; and migration, social change and development. The aged is her most recent area of research interest and a component of the family studies that have been her main focus in both population and migration studies.

Antonia Dalla Pria Bankoff holds a PhD in Morphofunctional Medicine (University of São Paulo), a graduate degree in Dentistry and under-graduate degree in Physical Education. She is Professor at the State University of Campinas, Brazil, and her research is on topics related to health and physical activity, electromyography, quality of life and obesity. She has been a Research Fellow and Visiting Professor to the University of Roma in Italy.

Sergio Bellantonio is Postdoctoral Research Fellow in General and Social Pedagogy at the Department of Physical Education, Sport and Wellness of the University of Naples *"Parthenope"* in Italy. His research interests include: educational approach to adolescence through sport activities with a special focus on corporeality and guidance, coping strategies in sports with emphasis on the body, and education and guidance in a constructivist and systemic perspective.

Bella Bello Bitugu is an Educationist and Sociologist with special focus on development and change. He holds a PhD from the University of Innsbruck in Austria, where he is still a guest lecturer. Since 2012, he has been the Director of the Sports Directorate of the University of Ghana, Legon. He is an expert in development through sport which uses the strength and power of sport to address development and other societal issues. He is also very involved in community projects and social development through sports in Africa and Europe. He works on the boards of FIFA, the United Nations Office for Sport and Peace Development, and several other European, African and American organizations.

Norma Angélica Borbón is a doctoral student in the Sciences of Physical Culture program at the autonomous University of Nuevo León. She holds a Master's degree in Physical Training and works as a scholar at the State University of Sonora. She conducts research and teaches in the applied sport sciences. She has participated in national and international conferences and presentations, and has published articles in national magazines.

Pedro G. Carvalho has a PhD in Economics from the University of Beira Interior (Covilhã, Portugal). He has been a visiting scholar at the University of Illinois Urbana-Champaign, and is currently Dean of the Human and Social Sciences Faculty (UBI). His research includes applied economics, social network analysis, public policy and regional development, as well as impact assessment of sport events and sport and health public policies. He has numerous publications in peer-reviewed journals and book chapters, as well as published several books. He serves on the Executive Board of the International Council of Sport Science and Physical Education.

Rosa María Cruz Castruita is Teacher and Researcher in the Facultad de Organización Deportiva (FOD) at Universidad Autónoma de Nuevo León (UANL). She holds a Master's and doctorate degree in Nursing Sciences from UANL. She holds professional memberships in various national and international organizations, including SHAPE (US Society of Health and Physical Education) and American Society of Aging (ASA). She supervises Master's and doctoral theses and is on the editorial board of the scientific journal *Facultad de Organización Deportiva (FOD)*. Her publications include over 20 scientific research articles.

Oswaldo Ceballos-Gurrola is President of the Latin American Association of Sport Science, Physical Education and Dance and was Dean of the School of Sport Organization. He earned his doctorate degree in Physical Activity and Sport Science at University of Zaragoza from Spain. He also studied three Master's degrees in Physical Education and Sport Management. He is the actual Vice President of the Board of Directors of the Mexican Association of Physical Culture Higher Education Institutions and member of National System of Researchers of the National Council of Science and Technology (CONACYT). He also belongs to the research group named Physical Culture and Sports Science. He has published 12 books and 8 chapters of different books printed by prestigious publishing houses, and has had more than 30 scientific articles published, some of them on physical activity for older adults.

Magdalena Soledad Chavero is a PhD student in the School of Public Health and Nutrition at the Faculty of Physical Culture–Autonomous University of Chihuahua. Her Master's degree is in Physical Education and Sport Management at the School of Public Health and Nutrition of the Universidad Autónoma de Nuevo León. She is currently working on research projects on the development of functions of teaching, management and mentoring; and has held an administrative position in the School of Public Health and Nutrition at the Autonomous University of Nuevo León from 1992 to 2009.

Aldo M. Costa is Assistant Professor in the Department of Sport Sciences at the University of Beira Interior (UBI). His research focus is in the area of teaching and athletic performance, including exercise physiology, training and testing. He has published papers in peer-reviewed research journals and books. He is reviewer of several ISA-indexed journals. In 2014, he won an honorable mention in Sports Science (sports training category) by the Portuguese Olympic Committee. He is frequently invited to participate as scientific advisor by the Portuguese Swimming Federation in several community projects related to "aquatic readiness" in the Portuguese population and "talent identification and development." Currently he is also Vice-President of the Portuguese Swimming Coaches Association.

Antonia Cunti is Full Professor of General and Social Pedagogy at the Department of Physical Education, Sport and Wellness of the University of Naples *"Parthenope"* in Italy. Her research interests are: (1) the education of human movement and sport and the relation among education, body and identity; and (2) educators' training in a reflective and systemic perspective, including counseling, educational cure and guidance processes. As head, she is responsible for the teachers' training courses and of guidance and counseling services at the same university.

Malathie P. Dissanayake is Senior Lecturer in Psychology at the Department of Psychology and Medical Psychology, Faculty of Medicine, South Asian Institute of Technology and Medicine (SAITM), Sri Lanka. At present she is the Head of the Department of Psychology and Medical Psychology. She holds a PhD in Developmental Psychology from North Carolina State University, USA, MA in General Psychology from West Chester University of Pennsylvania, USA, and BA (Hons) in Psychology from University of Peradeniya, Sri Lanka. She serves as a committee member of The Research Committee, The Medical Education Unit, and The Curriculum Development and Evaluation Committee, in the Faculty of Medicine, SAITM. She has won awards for her research and academic performance.

Eliana Lucia Ferreira has a PhD (2003) and Master's degree (1998) in Physical Education from UNICAMP. She is Professor at the Faculty of Physical Education (UFJF), Coordinator of the Accessibility Program, the long distance learning program and the research group of inclusion in the long distance learning NGIME/UFJF, since 2009. Currently, she has a position of trust in the Department of Continuing Education at the Ministry of Education, and is the representative of Brazil in the International Association of Physical Education and Sport for Girls and Women (IAPESGW) as well as a member of the International Council of Sport Science and Physical Education (ICSSPE).

Maria Beatriz Rocha Ferreira holds a PhD in Anthropology (University of Texas, 1987), and a Master's Degree in Physical Education (University of São Paulo, 1981). She has been a Research Fellow and Visiting Professor at universities in the USA, Belgium and Brazil. Her research topics include culture and society emphasizing diversity, figuration, power, gender, games and physical activity in different populations, such as indigenous peoples, Bolivians in the city of São Paulo, river dwellers called "ribeirinhos" in Amazonas and in wheelchair dance sport. She is a member of the Development Committee of the International Council of Sport Science and Physical Education.

Ludmila Fialova is Professor in the Department of Psychology, Pedagogy and Didactics in the Faculty of Physical Education and Sports at Charles University Prague, Czech Republic. She specializes in "Body image as a part in self-conception" and "School sport didactics." Her research deals with different aspects of Health Education, individual well-being and sport in local Czech and international context. She is author of 6 monographs, chapters in 13 monographs (11 abroad) and more than 200 vocational articles (in four languages – Czech, German, Russian and English). She participated in more than 20 research projects and international cooperation (with Germany, Russia, France and Poland).

María Dolores González-Rivera is Professor in the Department of Biomedical Science at University of Alcalá/Spain. She has published extensively on sport and physical activity professionals, gerontology and gender. Her publications include more than 60 articles, 1 book as well as 15 book chapters. In addition, she has participated in seven research projects, four of them funded by the Government of Spain. She is the reviewer of six journals. Furthermore, she has directed four doctoral theses and she is now directing five doctoral theses.

Ilse Hartmann-Tews is Full Professor and Head of the Department of Sociology and Gender Studies at the German Sport University Cologne. She has published intensively on gender issues in sport and on social structural aspects of ageing and sport (Hartmann-Tews, I., Tischer, U. & Conbrink, C. (2012) Bewegtes Alter(n). Sozialstrukturelle Aspekte von Sport und Alter(n). Opladen: Budrich). She is a member of the editorial board of the *International Review for the Sociology of Sport* (Sage) and of the *International Journal of Sport Policy and Politics* (Routledge). She was Dean of the Faculty of Social Sciences and is now a member of the Board of Directors of the German Sport University Cologne.

Marta Cañizares Hernández is Full Professor of Sports Psychology with a PhD in Psychological Sciences and Director of the Center for the Study of the Psychology of Physical Activity and Sports of the Universidad de Ciencias de la Cultura Física "Manuel Fajardo." She is the author of several books on psychology of sport and physical activity, and has lectured at many national and international scientific events, including: Brazil, Puerto Rico, Venezuela, Colombia, Ecuador, Mexico, France and Italy. She directs Master's and Doctoral theses and is in charge of the Master's program in Sport Psychology.

Urbano Ramiro Cañizares Hernández, who helped translate this chapter, is an English as Second Language (ESL) teacher who has collaborated with the author before. He graduated with a degree in English as a foreign language from Instituto Superior Pedagogico Felix Varela in Santa Clara, Cuba.

Maryam Koushkie Jahromi is Associate Professor in the Department of Sport Sciences Department at Shiraz University, in Iran. She holds a PhD in exercise physiology and her research focuses on physiological influences of exercise/sport/physical activity on women's health. Her research interests include: Muslim women's sport, and exercise/physical activities for children and the elderly. She has published over 55 articles and 8 books with national and international publishers and is an editorial board member of national and international journals. She has been an executive board member of IAPESGW from 2009–2017.

Rosa Olivia Méndez has a PhD from Instituto Tecnológico de Veracruz, Mexico. She works in the Research Center for Food and Development A.C., Hermosillo, Sonora. Mexico. Her research interest is in the area of mineral composition and nutritive value of food, and the nutritional status of iron, calcium and zinc in women. She works on the quantification of food and in the estimation of its availability using an in vitro method, and participates in projects that include the measurement of bone mass and body composition in children, youth and adults. She has evaluated the nutritional status of calcium and iron in women of childbearing age and postmenopausal stage. For the evaluation of the nutritional status of zinc, she has measured its absorption using stable isotopes and the expression of different zinc transporters (ZIP and ZnT) in adolescents.

Yael Netz is Professor in Gerontology at Wingate College of Physical Education and Sport Sciences in Israel. She is President of the European Group for Research into Elderly and Physical Activity – EGREPA and Co-editor in Chief of the *European Review of Aging and Physical Activity – EURAPA*. She has established the area of specialty on "Physical activity for older adults" at Wingate College and served, for many years, as the Head of this program. Her research has centered on the effect of various physical activity programs on physical, cognitive and emotional functioning in old and middle-aged populations, especially in Israel. She has dozens of publications in refereed journals and appears regularly at international conferences, at times as the keynote speaker. Recently, she is working on a project supported by Erasmus funding looking at balance and stability, developing health programs for healthy and frail elderly in Europe.

Reginald Ocansey is Director of the Research and Education Center at the Active Living & Wellness Alliance Group, Nungua, Ghana and part-time Emeritus Professor of Physical Activity Education and Research at the University of Education, Winneba, Ghana. He holds degrees from the Alabama State University and his doctorate from Ohio State University, USA. His research focuses on physical education, healthy kids and building an environment for physical activity. He has presented and published widely on these topics at national and international levels.

Martha Ornelas is Full Professor and Investigator at the Autonomous University of Chihuahua in Faculty of Physical Activity and Sport Sciences. She holds a PhD in Physical Activity and Health from the University of Granada. Her undergraduate and graduate degrees are in the field of Sport Psychology from the Autonomous University of Chihuahua, and her post-doctorate work was completed in the field of Human Sciences at the University of Zulia. She has presented research papers and published numerous studies. Since 2014, she has been a member of the National System of Researchers (SNI).

Rita Palmeira-de-Oliveira has a PhD in Pharmaceutical Sciences from the University of Beira Interior (UBI) and is Assistant Professor at the Faculty of Health Sciences at UBI. She supervises Master's and PhD students in Pharmaceutical Sciences and Biomedicine. She is also one of the owners of a spinoff company, Labfit, that is located at Ubimedical, and is a Hospital Pharmacist Specialist recognized by the Portuguese Pharmacists College. Her research areas are vaginal drug delivery systems, probiotics, essential oils and plant extracts, patient safety, medication reconciliation and potentially inappropriate medication for the elderly. She has been awarded prizes from the Portuguese Association of Hospital Pharmacists for her research on the implementation of medication reconciliation tools and a project to improve the prescription of drugs for the elderly. Her publications include 22 papers in international peer-reviewed journals, 3 book chapters and 4 patents (1 national, 3 international) and she was theme editor of a special issue on "Vaginal Drug Delivery" in the journal *Advanced Drug Delivery Reviews*.

Ana Pereira has a PhD in Science and Sport from the University of Tras-os-Montes and Alto Douro in Portugal. She is Co-coordinator of the Centre of Education and Research Training of the Polytechnic Institute of Setubal and an Adjunct Professor in the School of Education. She has published over 40 articles and presented more than 80 research papers nationally and internationally. She also supervises Master's and doctoral theses.

Elizabeth Raymond is a graduate student in the Psychology Department of West Chester University of Pennsylvania. She has been a Research Assistant to Dr. Tahmaseb McConatha and has worked on several research projects in the area of Gender and Gerontology, which have led to five presentations (peer-reviewed) and six manuscript publications.

Nancy Cristina Banda Sauceda has a Master's in Exercise Sciences (2012) focusing on High-Performance Athletes and an undergraduate degree in Nutrition (2002) from the Autonomous University of Nuevo León (UANL). Her research focuses on the impact of exercise and sport on the body as well as the influence of nutrition.

Introduction

Karin Volkwein-Caplan and
Jasmin Tahmaseb McConatha

Introduction

The world is aging. The population of older adults is expanding exponentially. By the year 2050 experts predict that one-third of the world's population will be over 60 years of old (www.ilcusa.org). In the next 40 years, in the United States alone the number of older men and women (over the age of 65) is projected to double from 46 million to 98 million. Throughout the world, older adults are also becoming more ethnically and racially diverse. Although maximal life expectancy has changed little over the centuries, average life expectancy has increased from 49 at the turn of the twentieth century to almost 80 in industrialized nations at the turn of the twenty-first century. A longevity gender gap also continues. In all countries women not only continue to outnumber men but live longer lives. Studies have found that perhaps half of the variance in longevity can be associated with genetic factors. Personal, social, and cultural factors account for the remaining influences on how long a person can expect to live. There are numerous factors that contribute to a long and healthy life. How well one is able to successfully engage in health promoting activities, such as exercise or fitness activities, is an important component of later life health and well-being.

An individual's sense of well-being is also affected by the interacting effects of genetic heritage, economic circumstances, social relationships, emotional bonds, cultural values, personality traits and spiritual beliefs. Resources such as access to health care and to nature also have an impact of later life well-being. These, of course, vary significantly from country to country. The major factors that threaten well-being in the twenty-first century are significantly different for elders in industrialized countries than for those in non-industrialized societies. In some parts of the world, the spread of infectious diseases, the absence of sanitation, the difficulty of maintaining personal hygiene, deficient diet, and limited access to quality medical care are still major threats to the health and well-being of older adults. The ability to engage in health promoting behaviors such as exercise is also influenced by social conditionals such as political turmoil.

Expectations for a "healthy" later adulthood vary culturally. In some societies, older men and women continue to work. They travel and continue their educations. In other societies elders look forward to a time of rest and relaxation after a lifetime of work that may well have involved strenuous physical activity. Regardless of personal circumstances, it is clear that health concerns and health promotion are very much in the thoughts of older men and women. Older adults, of course, require more long-term medical services than any other portion of the population. Given the growing number of older adults, it becomes increasingly important to address health behaviors and lifestyles that affect their sense of well-being. This anthology is a snapshot of the factors influencing the well-being of older men and women.

Health promotion for elders is an increasingly important topic for social and political planning. (www.census.gov). Numerous studies have found that staying physically active leads to increased well-being and happiness in older adulthood (Tahmaseb McConatha & Volkwein-Caplan, 2010; Volkwein & McConatha, 2012; Volkwein-Caplan, 2014). People who are physically and socially active seem to be most likely to maintain their physical and psychological health (Volkwein & McConatha, 2012). It is therefore critical that older adults have access to places and spaces in which they can be active, an access that would ensure a more graceful and healthy aging process.

The centrality of fitness in the successful aging model also devolves from a person's degree of social and community support and the all-important availability of resources (fitness facilities, walking trails, organized activities) that enable physical activity. The international experts who have contributed essays to this collection describe the in-country status of health promotion outreach programs, best practices packages, and promotional campaigns that underscore the physical and psychological importance of physical activity.

Exercise, physical activity, health, and longevity

Classical philosophers, doctors, researchers, and scientists have long claimed that exercise and physical activity is a miracle drug in the anti-aging process. Given that the world is graying, more and more has been published on this issue. Indeed, due to scientific, technological, and medical advances, life expectancy has increased exponentially across the globe. The expansion of the older adult population is both a burden and an opportunity.

In 2017 *Time Magazine* devoted a special edition to "The Science of Exercise" and the year before an issue on "The Exercise Cure." Numerous studies have addressed the importance of physical and social activity across the life-span. Although exercise has been associated with increased well-being and longevity, we also know that the majority of older men and women in the world do not engage in regular exercise.

What is the current status in research and how can we best prepare for this socio-psycho-medical phenomenon of aging? This book will attempt to answer some of these pressing questions, provide examples of what works in the respective countries of the authors, and what still needs to happen so that we might be prepared to assist the aging population adequately in the near future. How can we move from "sick" care to a "health" care? In this volume, the contributors discuss programs in which countries, communities, and organizations have attempted to promote the well-being of older adults through the promotion of services and education programs that can lead to increased activity and subsequently improved health and well-being.

Can exercise indeed be used as a medicine for the old and sick? Exercise physiologists have incontrovertible proof that exercise and physical activity improves the quality and duration of life. Physicians who have prescribed exercise to their patients have found "that even walking, anything that gets their heart rate up a bit results in the dramatic improvement of chronic disease, depression, anxiety, mood and energy levels—but only if it is done on a regular basis" (Oaklander, 2016, 60). Studies in which blood has been drawn right after individuals have exercised show that positive changes occur throughout the body during and right after the activity. "It's unbelievable. If there were a drug that could do for human health everything that exercise can, it would likely be the most valuable pharmaceutical ever developed" (Oaklander, 2016, 56).

Despite the overwhelming evidence that addresses the health benefits associated with regular activity, studies indicate that the majority of older adults do not engage in even the minimum required physical activity levels. In fact, only 20 percent of people in North America get the recommended 150 minutes of exercise per week, including strength and cardio-vascular physical activity. And half of all baby-boomers (age 65+) do not exercise. And yet we know that a body in motion is very healthy. Consider these amazing facts (Oaklander, 2016):

- Moving quickly makes the heart pump more blood to the body's tissue, including the muscle. Extra oxygen makes muscle better combat fatigue.
- Repeated weight-bearing contractions make muscles grow and put pressure on the bones, increasing their density.
- Increased blood flow to the brain creates new blood vessels. Exercise also creates the release of chemicals in the body that dull pain and lighten mood.

- Exercise may protect telomeres, thus, slowing down the aging of cells.
- The body is better able to burn fat for energy, causing fat cells to shrink.
- Exercise increases blood flow to the skin helping wounds to heal faster.

Exercise does not only stimulate the heart, muscle, lungs, and bones, but also the brain. This fact is very important for the older generation. Indeed, regular exercise has been shown to prevent or delay the onset of chronic conditions such as heart disease, cancer, diabetes, and even Alzheimer's disease. Thus, engaging in any kind of physical activity contributes to the restoration of the body, which, in turn, slows down cellular aging. The majority of older men and women are not aware of the multiple benefits of exercise. Some of them who may be struggling with depression may lack the motivation or the resources to engage in regular activity.

What can the readers expect?

As is the case with all books from the International Council of Sport and Physical Education (ICSSPE), this book seeks to bring together insights and experiences from around the world. The international array of contributors to this book considers the importance of exercise and physical activity in later life. In their chapters, they present an overview of programs, services, research, as well as the health promoting factors that have led to increased physical activity levels in older men and women in their respective countries. Furthermore, the centrality of fitness in the successful aging model is addressed from a person's degree of social and community support as well as the all-important availability of resources (fitness facilities, walking trails, organized activities) that promote physical activity. Our group of international experts, including scholars from North and South America, Eastern and Western Europe, Asia, Africa, as well as the Middle and Far East, write about their particular health promotion outreach programs, best care practices packages, and promotional campaigns—programs that underscore the physical and psychological importance of physical activity. More specifically, the contributors focus on the following themes and link them to the aging, fitness, and sports programs in their particular nations:

- health promotion (history, current status, future plans/needs);
- health and longevity;
- chronic illness;
- fitness, nutrition, sports;
- social and mental health programs;
- health education;

- inequities (gender, social class, ethnicity, health) of access to health and fitness resources.

These themes shape the organizational structure of each chapter. The chapters are organized into three parts. Part I chapters are general overviews of the importance of culture, community, and the impact of well-being in the aging process. Part II contributions focus on the effects of physical activity and exercise on the aging population. Finally, the Part III chapters describe with precision how physical movement enables many elders to cope with the burdens of chronic illnesses.

Part I begins with the analysis of the importance of the socio-cultural environment, specifically the place and space in which one lives and its impact on the aging process. Chapter 1 provides examples of healthy aging in so-called age-friendly communities in the USA. These include opportunities for civic engagement and criteria for promoting safety, physical activity, healthy nutrition, and combating ageism. Chapter 2 describes images of aging and physical activity of elderly in Germany, focusing on active aging discourses over the last 20 years. The impact of gender and social class are analyzed as they are represented in who is engaging in physical activity and what exercises are preferred by the elderly. Chapter 3 describes the design and implementation of new policies and approaches concerning exercise and physical activity as important instruments to support healthy aging in Portugal. The power of sports in society—including the support of health prevention, social peace, and ethical decision making—plays a key role in the implementation of an official framework to combat premature aging and increase the overall quality of life for older adults. Chapter 4 spells out the high risk of decreasing functional capacity of the elderly as a result of changes due to the bio-psycho-social aging process. The role of active aging is addressed as it applies to elders in Mexico and Latin America. The chapter discusses how maintaining autonomy and suggesting behavioral change charts a path toward health. Chapter 5 discusses the current situation of aging in Ghana from a cultural and public health perspective. Traditional norms that have supported healthy aging and provided a safety net are being rapidly transformed by increasing urbanization and migration. Emerging formal care systems are therefore expected to complement the traditional debilitated norms. Best practices for the future that suit the local norms and culture are developed.

Part II focuses specifically on the role and effects of physical activity and exercise on the aging population. Chapter 6 lays out principles and practices of healthy aging in Brazil and describes the risk factors associated with an inactive lifestyle, the absence of adequate facilities, and resistance to behavior change. Chapter 7 provides excellent examples of healthy aging practiced in Cuba and its effect on the physical and mental health status of the elderly in general as well as former athletes. Chapter 8 describes how fitness programs influence and intervene with the general decline as people get older in Spain. Socio-cultural barriers, resources, and social conditions present challenges for adequate responses to the needs of older adults. Chapter 9 provides insights on the changing health care system and the comprehension of the physical self in the Czech Republic. It focuses on the importance of an active lifestyle and health promotion on the well-being of the elderly and reviews programs and practices in place. Chapter 10 considers the physical practices established for the older population in Israel and analyzes how activity affects the psychological functioning, longevity, loneliness, and social interactions of this age group. Chapter 11 presents the role and status of physical activity, its barriers and facilitators in Iranian elderly people's life.

Part III describes an array of chronic conditions with which older people have to cope. How does the impact of physical activity and exercise influence their well-being? Chapter 12 spells out the coping mechanisms of chronic illness in the USA. Illness management includes healthy lifestyle factors such as exercise, diet, and stress management. Chapter 13 studies the role of education impacting engagement in physical activity and health in Italy. The impact of "Mature Sports Clubs" as well as various formal and non-formal community and health education strategies are analyzed regarding the promotion of physical activity and health. Chapter 14 looks into South Asian best practices for achieving active and healthy aging in Sri Lanka. It considers the challenges presented by health complications and disability among the elderly.

The conclusion synthesizes what can be learned from failures and best practices established throughout the world. It provides a future perspective on active and healthy aging across the world. The insights gained from our global perspective on aging direct us to a felicitous path that can guide us toward a future of elderly health and well-being

Note: Throughout this text authors from different parts of the world are referring to ageing OR aging, which is both correct. The same is true for describing older people as elderly or the aged, referring generally to the age group 60+ or 65+. Hence, the editors left these fine details for each chapter intact, since they also seemed country-specific.

References

Oaklander, M. (2016). The New Science of Exercise. *Time Magazine, 188* (10–11), 54–60.

Tahmaseb McConatha, J. & Volkwein-Caplan, K. (2010). *Cultural Contours of the Body: Aging and Fitness*. Dubuque, IA: Kendall-Hunt, USA.

Time Magazine. (August, 2017). Special Issue: *The Science of Exercise*.

Volkwein, K. & McConatha, J. (2012). *The Social Geography of Healthy Aging*. Aachen, Germany: Meyer & Meyer Publishers.

Volkwein-Caplan, K. (2014). *Sport|Fitness|Culture*. London: Meyer & Meyer Sport.

Part I

Importance of culture, community, and the impact of well-being in the aging process

The social and cultural context of well-being and physical activity in later life in the USA

Jasmin Tahmaseb McConatha,
Karin Volkwein-Caplan, and
Amarachi Akwarandu

Introduction

The number of adults over the age of 65 makes up 8 percent of the world's population (NIH, 2015). In the U.S. older adults, aged 65 and older, represented 14.1 percent of the U.S. population in 2013. The older adult population is the fastest growing segment of North American society. It is estimated that by the year 2035, 20 percent (70 million) of the population of the United States will be 65 and older, a significant increase from 1900 when older adults made up 4 percent of the population (www.census.gov). As the U.S. population ages, it becomes increasingly important to address factors that impact the health and well-being of older men and women. Promoting and maintaining well-being in later life must be approached holistically from a physical, mental, spiritual, social, and community perspective. As the older adult population grows, an increasing number of cities and communities are striving to better meet the needs of their older adult residents. This chapter outlines examples of community services and resources that help older adults live healthy, active, and independent lives.

Social and cultural context of well-being and physical activity in later life

The ways in which an increasing population of older adults attempts to maintain health and well-being cannot be separated from the communities and cultures in which they live. In 2010, The World Health Organization (WHO) established the WHO Global Network of Age-friendly Cities and Communities (WHO, 2016). This global network connects organizations, communities, and cities that have the goal of providing their residents with a safe and comfortable place to grow old. The communities involved in this global network make a commitment to assess, monitor, and whenever possible develop services and resources for older adults. While community assessment and development takes a number of different forms, the eight components listed below are of essential importance. These domains provide the communities with opportunities to plan for improvement in physical and social engagements that can help increase the health and well-being of community residents:

1   opportunities for physical and social participation;
2   access to transportation;
3   affordable and safe housing;
4   outdoor spaces and buildings;
5   respect for diversity and social inclusion;
6   opportunities for civic participation and employment;
7   access to communication and information;
8   access to community services and health care.

As the WHO, the American Associations of Retired Persons (AARP), and other organizations have recognized, no one can age well alone. Each person's well-being is imbedded in a network of community, society, and culture. A person's well-being is dependent upon the ways in which people have available and make use of physiological, social, and environmental resources which help them maintain competencies as they age (McConatha, McConatha, & Dermigny, 1994; McConatha, McConatha, Deaner, & Dermigny, 1995; Pavot & Diener, 2004; Krause, 2010). Numerous researchers (Tahmaseb McConatha, 2013; Volkwein & McConatha, 2014; Haselwandter, Corcoran, Folta, Hyatt, Fenton, & Nelson, 2015) have indicated that the physical and social environment has a direct link to a person's health and happiness in later life. They enable and promote more active and healthy lifestyles. Parks, Senior Centers, community centers, sidewalks, and farmers markets are a few examples of community resources that have been found to promote a more active and healthy aging experience. Addressing factors which promote the well-being and happiness of aging men and women can have significant humanistic and economic consequences. Older adults with greater economic, instrumental, social, and cultural resources are happier, healthier, and more satisfied with life. Community resources can serve a buffering function helping older men and women cope with the stressors associated with health related concerns in later life.

Support and well-being in later life

Researchers (Tulle, 2008; Volkwein & McConatha, 2012) have indicated that social integration and physical activity are two of the most important factors determining health and well-being in later adulthood (Tahmaseb McConatha & DiGregorio, 2007; Volkwein & McConatha, 2012). Active engagement in life has been associated with a multitude of positive consequences (Volkwein-Caplan, 2014). Older adults who are able to stay active and maintain a sense of integration and connection with their families and communities have been shown to experience fewer chronic illnesses and experience less unhappiness, dissatisfaction, isolation, anxiety, and depression.

Exercise bolsters self-esteem, increases life satisfaction, and improves overall feelings of well-being. Whether or not older adults exercise is dependent upon a number of interrelated factors including education, ethnicity, health concerns, as well as socioeconomic status (Tahmaseb McConatha & Volkwein-Caplan, 2010). Given the strength of the relationships between exercise and well-being, it is surprising that the majority of older Americans do not participate in regular exercise. Perhaps one reason for this lack of activity is the lack of availability of places and programs for elders to engage in physical activity.

Investigators (Haselwandter, Corcoran, Folta, Hyatt, Fenton, & Nelson, 2015) have recently found that only about one-quarter, clearly a small percentage of older Americans aged 60 and above, exercise regularly. The lack of environmental support is one of the reasons for this low activity rate. The "built environment" needs to provide the places and spaces that will motivate activity (Haselwandter, Corcoran, Folta, Hyatt, Fenton, & Nelson, 2015). The built environment can be described as the "physical environment in which an individual spends his or her time; it includes sidewalks, parks, crosswalks, and manageable traffic patterns, among other factors" (Haselwandter, Corcoran, Folta, Hyatt, Fenton, & Nelson, 2015, p. 323). Older adults whose built environment consists of features that allow or even require them to stay physically active tend to have higher overall physical activity levels than older adults who do not live in such environments.

There are a number of social and psychological factors which impact activity level in later life as well. One of the most important risk factors that contributes to a reduced quality of life and mortality in older adults is depression (Holmquist, Mattsson, Schele, Nordstrom, & Nordstrom, 2016). Seven percent of older adults ages 60 and above suffer from depression; however, these statistics are significantly underestimated given that most mental health concerns in later life are both under diagnosed and undertreated (WHO, 2016). According to Holmquist et al. (2016), low levels of physical functioning in everyday life have been associated with an increase in psychological disorders such as depression as well as medical conditions such as diabetes and poorer health status in general. By contrast, engaging in physical activities has been proven to have preventative and beneficial effects on depressive symptoms within older adults.

In order to illustrate the importance of the relationship between activity and well-being in later life, this chapter addresses community support and barriers that promote or hinder physical activity patterns among older

Americans. In addition, psychological factors play and integral role on the overall well-being of the individual, and they can either promote or hinder participation in physical activity.

Quality of life and physical activity

As stated above, regular physical activity or exercise is an important factor influencing health and well-being (Katz, 2000; Tulle, 2008). Exercise may involve simple activities such as walking, jogging, stretching, or a variety of other more complex activities, including yoga, recreational, or various sport activities. Researchers have even framed the term *functional fitness*, which includes any form of physical activity that people perform in their daily lives, i.e., walking to the grocery store and carrying the load back home up the stairs (Volkwein-Caplan, 2014). The physical and psychological benefits of exercise have been well documented: exercise bolsters self-esteem, increases life satisfaction, and improves overall feelings of well-being (Katz, 2000; Tulle, 2008; Volkwein-Caplan, 2014). Exercise also influences several components of overall self-image, including body image and self-efficacy or one's belief that one is able to exercise, self-esteem, feelings of control, and life satisfaction. Self-efficacy, for example, has been shown to lead to feelings of competence and physical acceptance; older adults gain confidence in their overall physical and psychological abilities through exercise (Sonstroem & Potts, 1996).

Exercise and recreational activities have the potential to be positively related to control, independence, decision making, physical and social involvement, stress reduction, and feelings of hopefulness about life in general. Active older adults also rated their self- reported health as better and had lower depression scores than those that were inactive (Volkwein-Caplan, 2014). By contrast, older adults who do not engage in regular exercise were found to be more depressed, more anxious, and less satisfied with their life (Holmquist, Mattsson, Schele, Nordstrom, & Nordstrom, 2016). Inactive older adults also had lower self-rated health and developed more physical illnesses than the active older adults (Tahmaseb McConatha & Volkwein-Caplan, 2010). They have also been found to decline in their functional fitness level or the ability to engage in everyday activities competently.

Predictors of exercise behavior in older adults

A number of factors predict whether or not someone exercises. Analysis of population health and well-being across the United States indicates that there are significant variations, for example location and community are key factors. The healthiest states in the U.S. tend to be located in New England, Vermont, Massachusetts, New Hampshire, and Connecticut, although Hawaii appears to be the healthiest. The unhealthiest by contrast are located in the South, Mississippi, Louisiana, and Alabama tend to have less healthy lifestyles, poorer air quality, higher levels of smoking and drinking, and lower levels of physical activity (WHO, 2016).

Clearly community is a key factor influencing health. Healthier adults are more likely to exercise (Tulle, 2008). Ethnicity, gender, and social class also influence exercise participation. For example, differences have been identified in the exercise patterns of African Americans and European Americans. Studies have suggested that older African American adults engage in less physical activity than their White counterparts. Researchers speculate the lack of physical activity in later life may be a result of the fact that many African Americans had earlier occupations that involved physical activity and, therefore, perceive physical activity as related to "work" (Jones, 2007).

Older adults from a lower socioeconomic background tend to be less active than middle and upper class adults. Shutzer and Graves (2004) speculate that a lack of resources, such as membership to health clubs and the availability of facilities, in combination with a background of physical labor may explain the lack of exercise. Gender differences have also been found in the exercise patterns of older adults (Twigg, 2004). For example, Felton, Parsons, and Bartoces (1997) found that men engage in more exercise activities than women. The authors also found that men and women have different ideas of what constitutes exercise. For example, men reported participation in more formal exercise and in sport, whereas women tended to see involvement with family activities and even household chores as exercise.

Education, ethnicity, cultural values and norms, as well as socioeconomic factors interact and influence physical activities (Elavsky et al., 2005). Older adults may be unaware of the importance of regular physical activity or they may fear injury or health risks if they exercise. Those who live in poverty stricken or unsafe neighborhoods and communities without access to parks, clubs, and other places to exercise are clearly at a disadvantage when it comes to being able to find ways to stay physically active, even if they wish to do so.

Senior Centers and other community resources and the promotion of physical activity

Community resources such as Senior Centers connect older adults to vital community services that can assist them in staying healthy and independent. Senior Centers provide a variety of services for older adults, such as transportation, health and fitness programs, employment assistance, social and recreational activities, intergenerational programs, meal and nutrition programs, volunteer and civic engagement opportunities, and educational and arts programs. Older adults who utilize Senior Center services have higher levels of social interaction, physical activity, and life satisfaction.

Senior Centers are widespread around the United States. Membership costs to centers are generally very low (10 to 25 dollars a year) and centers tend to offer transportation. Senior Centers are, therefore, a source of support, a place that can provide space and opportunity for older adults from diverse backgrounds to exercise. Members of the Senior Center are community residing older adults who attend activities of interest to them at the Center. Senior Centers have developed in order to provide a source of community support for older adults. These centers provide friendship, activities, education, and nourishment. They tend to offer a variety of programs including exercise classes, yoga, intergenerational programs, language classes, trips, spiritual discussions, current events, crafts, line dancing, and computer classes, to name only a few.

In a recent community assessment, 579 participants over the age of 60, who were members of a local Senior Center responded to surveys of well-being and an assessment of physical activity (Tahmaseb McConatha, forthcoming). The study focused on an investigation of the exercise pattern of a group of older adults who were members and regular attendees of a local Senior Center. The results indicated that participants who visited the Senior Center regularly and engaged in group exercises were significantly more likely to exercise outside of the Center than the general population of adults over the age of 65. Almost 60 percent of participants stated that they exercise at least three times a week for a minimum of 30 minutes. Most participants exercised for at least 60 minutes four to five times a week. In this study we also explored the relationship between exercise and self-esteem, life satisfaction, control, and self-efficacy. Analysis indicated that participants who engaged in exercise generally scored high on these dimensions of well-being. In short, those who participated in Senior Center activities were more likely to exercise while at the Center but also at other times; and those who exercised were more likely to have higher levels of life satisfaction, higher feelings of self-esteem and self-efficacy, and greater feelings of control over their lives. Of course it may be that more active older adults also are more likely to attend Senior Center functions. The majority of the people in this particular community assessment project, however, stated the participation in activities at the Center also motivated them to walk, garden, and stay active at other times.

Consistent with this finding, previous researchers focusing on the well-being of older adults have indicated that available community support promotes both physical and psychological benefits for older adults (Tahmaseb McConatha & Volkwein-Caplan, 2010). It has been indicated that only 25 to 33 percent of older adults in the United States engage in regular exercise. Over 60 percent of the older adult population do not exercise regularly, and 31 percent do not exercise at all (Shutzer & Graves, 2004). Clearly, a supportive community influences the exercise patterns of older Americans. If Senior Center participation has such a significant influence on the well-being of older adults, it would appear that the well-being of older adults can be bolstered by community programs which offer opportunity and space to exercise and socialize.

Participation in a Senior Center may lead to more physical activity, involvement in community, and subsequently greater health and well-being. Researchers such as Havighurst (1972) have suggested that more active older adults report higher levels of well-being, control, life satisfaction, self-esteem, and self-efficacy. This theory proposes that older adults substitute new social roles and responsibilities for the ones they leave behind, and that those older adults who maintain high social activity levels are the most satisfied and better adjusted than less active older adults.

As the example above illustrates, there is a dynamic relationship between the ways in which the social environment views aging and the quality of the aging experience. Community resources influence a sense of competence in older adults, which impacts motivation for physical and social activity. A lack of competence, on the other hand, has been associated with lower self-esteem, life satisfaction, and greater use of home health care services, greater risk of hospitalization and institutionalization and higher mortality. Activities that are meaningful to the maintenance of a positive sense of self enhance well-being in later adulthood. Productive activities and culturally meaningful activities are particularly effective in maintaining a positive and/or competent sense of self regardless of age.

Person-environmental fit model

The *person-environmental fit model* (Kahana, 1982) focuses on the "fit" of an individual's competence relative to demands of the physical environment. According to Kahana, the quality of life in later adulthood is largely dependent upon the interaction between a person's characteristics and the demands and resources of their environment. If the challenges and demands of the environment are significantly above or significantly below an individual's capabilities, a decline in well-being, feelings of control and competence, learned helplessness, and depression may result. In general a "good fit" results when the environmental press slightly exceeds the competence level of the individual (Lawton, 1985). The environmental press can be managed by either altering the situational context (e.g., being placed in a situation where fewer demands are made on the individual) or by increasing individual competencies.

Positive changes in an individual's activity level can decrease the risk of physical and psychological disorders. The key to successful aging is to accept and adapt to age-related changes by developing and maintaining healthy behaviors and lifestyles. Community programs and professionals can assist older adults in aging successfully by providing opportunities for active engagement, by developing programs to educate and foster healthy behaviors and lifestyles such as regular exercise and social activity.

Through primary, secondary, and tertiary prevention, healthier and more active lifestyles can be promoted. Primary prevention focuses on education and awareness, secondary prevention can be accomplished through providing health prevention programs (i.e., free weekly blood pressure screenings) at aging and health services organizations such as Senior Centers, and tertiary prevention will focus on the development of healthier behaviors and lifestyles through their participation in the health promoting programs such as exercise classes. Exercise builds a positive self-concept, increases self-confidence, and strengthens the body. Exercise also provides a means for socialization, which has been found to have a positive effect on older adults' health status and perceptions of health.

Older adults who are in good health, remain active, and have positive social interactions, generally do not experience a great decline in their physical and cognitive abilities. Developing and maintaining healthy life-styles can increase independence and overall life satisfaction. Community resources, such as health promotion programs, can increase older adults' awareness that one of the consequences of unhealthy behaviors and life-styles can be a loss of health and even independence. As the number of older adults continues to grow renewed attention to the health and well-being of this population is an important consideration. Contemporary older adults have the opportunity to be healthier, happier, and more educated than previous generations. Social and cultural awareness of the physical and psychological benefits of exercise can result in a more active and health conscious older adult population. In turn, these benefits can increase feelings of well-being and life satisfaction.

Conclusion

There were 47.8 million people over the age of 65 in the United States in 2015, accounting for 14.9 percent of the population. The growth in the population of older adults has resulted in a corresponding increase in communities focusing on providing services for the promotion of health and well-being of this population. There are an increasing number of healthy lifestyle and residential choices available to older American men and women. These choices focus on community engagement and health promotion. Programs and services promote healthy aging by encouraging and providing opportunities for physical and social activity and encouraging independence.

Supportive communities help diminish the chance of chronic illness, with maintenance of cognitive and physical ability and the enhancement of active engagement with life. Given the increase in life expectancy, older men and women need to be able to evaluate their social, physical, and economic circumstances and make informed decisions about their day-to-day experiences. Accessibility to services, community, housing design, and friendships are health-enhancing factors. Neighborhoods that promote a sense of community belonging, well-being, and incorporate social activities as well as physical fitness accessibility can make a significant difference in the aging experience of residents. Physical fitness accessibility such as local parks, biking/running trails, community gardens, or fitness clubs are important aspects of "age friendly" communities—an environment which is conducive to social activity and physical fitness as well as promoting safety and well-being of residents of all ages.

Older adults can receive assistance and support in the community. This often influences where older adults reside and the services they receive. Since life expectancy is increasing globally and also in this country, maintaining optimum physical and mental health is an ever-present challenge for older adults. Even though modern medicine has reached many milestones in treating illnesses that affect older adults, there is a rise in obesity and diabetes. Chronic diseases can affect older adults in their daily functioning. It has to be mentioned that although the role of healthy eating has not been addressed in this chapter, it is also an important factor besides the environment and access to physical activity to ensure a healthy aging process.

Given the growing population of older adults in the United States, there is an increased demand for research focusing on the needs of this cohort. The increase in life expectancy creates a myriad of contemporary health care, residential, financial, and community planning concerns not experienced by earlier generations. The advocacy work of groups like the AARP and the WHO will have to change in order to better suit the needs of this age group. It is in society's best interest to consider the health needs of *all* of its population. Health is not just the absence of illness but also the promotion of happiness and life satisfaction. Supportive communities can aid older adults not only by physical, social, and emotional supports, but also promote personal well-being and psychological functioning.

References

Chong, S., Ng, S.-H., Woo, J., & Kwan, A. Y.-H. (2006). Positive aging: The views of middle-aged and older adults in Hong Kong. *Aging Society, 26*, 243–265.

Diener, E., Emmons, R.A., Larsen, R.J., & Griffin, S. (1985). The satisfaction with life scale. *Journal of Personality Assessment, 49*, 71–75.

Elavsky, S., McAuley, E., Motl, R.W., Konopack, J.F., Marquez, D.X., Hu, L., Gerald, J.J., & Diener, E. (2005). Physical activity enhances long-term quality of life in older adults: Efficacy, esteem, and affective influences. *The Society of Behavioral Medicine, 30*, 138–145.

Felton, G., Parsons, M.A., & Bartoces, M.G. (1997). Demographic factors: Inter-action effects on health promoting behavior and health related factors. *Public Health Nursing, 14*, 361–367.

Haselwandter, E.M., Corcoran, S., Folta, S.C., Hyatt, R., Fenton, M., & Nelson, M.E. (2015). The built environment, physical activity, and aging in the United States: A state of the science review. *Journal of Aging and Physical Activity, 23*, 323–329.

Havighurst, R.J. (1972). *Developmental tasks and education*. New York: McKay.

Holmquist, S., Mattsson, S., Schele, I., Nordstrom, P., & Nordstrom, A. (2016). Low physical activity as a key differentiating factor in the potential high-risk profile for depressive symptoms in older adults. *Depress Anxiety, 34*, 1–9.

Jones, M. (2007). The relationships of perceived benefits of and barriers to reported exercise in older African American women. *Public Health Nursing, 13*, 151–158.

Kahana, E. (1982). A congruence model of person-environment interaction. In M.P. Lawton, P. Windley, & T.O. Byerts (Eds.), *Aging and the environment: Theoretical approaches* (pp. 97–121). New York: Springer.

Katz, S. (2000). Busy bodies: Activity, aging, and the management of everyday life. *Journal of Aging Studies, 14*, 135–152.

Lawton, M.P. & Nahemow, L. (1973) Ecology and the aging process. In C. Eisdorfer & M.P. Lawton (Eds.), *The psychology of adult development and aging*. Washington, DC: American Psychological Association.

National Institute of Health (NIH). (2016). Retrieved from www.nih.gov.

Tahmaseb McConatha, J. & DiGregorio, N. (2007). A gender and cultural comparison of the relationship between free time and perceived quality of life. *The International Journal of the Humanities, 5*, 235–242.

Tahmaseb McConatha, J. & Volkwein-Caplan, K. (2010). *Cultural contours of the body: Aging and fitness*. Dubuque, IA: Kendall Hunt Publishers.

Rosenberg, M. (1965). *Society and the adolescent self-image*. Princeton, NJ: Princeton University Press.

Shutzer, K.A. & Graves, B.S. (2004). Barriers and motivations to exercise in older adults. *Preventative Medicine, 39*, 1056–1061.

Sonstroem, R.J. & Potts, S.A. (1996). Life adjustment correlates of physical self-concepts. *Medicine and Science in Sports and Exercise, 28*, 619–625.

Tulle, E. (2008). Acting your age? Sports science and the aging body. *Journal of Aging Studies, 22*, 340–347.

Twigg, J. (2004). The body, gender, and age: Feminist insights in social gerontology. *Journal of Aging Studies, 18*, 69–73.

United States Census Bureau. (2010). Retrieved from www.census.gov.

Volkwein-Caplan, K. (2014). *Sport|fitness|culture*. Aachen, Germany: Meyer & Meyer Sport Publishers.

Volkwein, K. & McConatha, J. (2012). *The social geography of healthy aging. The importance of place and space*. Aachen, Germany: Meyer & Meyer Sport Publishers.

World Health Organization (WHO). (2016). Retrieved from: www.who.int/ageing/age-friendly-world/en/.

Chapter 2

The active ageing paradigm and physical activity of older people in Germany

Ilse Hartmann-Tews

Introduction

Images of ageing have changed a lot over the past decades in Germany and the same holds true of the image of sports and physical activities. The chapter starts with a brief outline of these two developments that have evolved independently but are related to each other. The second part presents empirical data about the development of participation in sport and physical activities of the elderly with respect to cross-sectional and longitudinal studies and a focus on socio-structural influences. The final section sums up the results and puts them in the broader frame of social change and public discourses on ageing in Germany.

Sportification of society

Sport sociologists describe the development of sports and physical activities in Germany over the past decades as a process of sportification of society, a term that refers to three dimension of sport development. The first dimension is an increase in participation and diversity of people that have become physically active over the past decades. Forty years ago participating in sports was mainly the domain of young men of the middle and upper classes in Germany. Nowadays, physical activity and sport participation are wide-spread leisure activities performed and realized by a diverse range of people, young and old, men and women, and people with different social and ethnic backgrounds. The second dimension of sportification refers to the diversification of sports and physical activities. In Germany up to the 1970s, sports were meant to be competitive and performance oriented with training regimes in sports clubs. Over the past decades, manifold new physical activities and hybrid forms of sporting activities have been invented. This development is mirrored in the development of a variety of new terms indicating the multifarious meanings attached to physical activities and sport, such as leisure-sport, adventure-sport, endurance-sport, trend-sport, alternative-sport, health and wellness-sport, rehabilitation, cardio, and fitness sports.

The third dimension complements this semantic broadening of the meanings of sport as there has been an increase in providers of physical activities and sport. Single and multisport clubs at grass root level are still the main provider of sport and physical activities in Germany. In the 1970s there were about 39,000 sports clubs with 10.1 million memberships. In 2017, there are about 90,000 voluntary-run sports clubs with about 27 million memberships. However, there have been a growing number of commercial providers for individual sports like tennis, squash, gymnastics, climbing, fitness, and yoga. Whereas the number of sports clubs and memberships is stagnating, the commercial fitness sector is still increasing and comprises about 7,000 centers with about 7 million customers. Besides this institutionalized form of sport and exercise participation, people have also increasingly entered natural spaces to engage in their sports individually without being a member of a sports club or a customer of a commercial provider. The term sportification of society therefore nicely reflects the realization of the idea of the European Charta Sport for All, developed in the 1960s (Hartmann-Tews, 1998).

Against this backdrop, the question arises with respect to an ageing society: Are elderly people part of this sportification process? To answer this question, a brief outline of the discourses on age(ing) in Germany will frame the analysis of the empirical studies conducted about the involvement of older people in sport and physical activities.

Public discourse on age(ing) and image shift of ageing in Germany

There has been a demographic shift in Germany toward the so-called "ageing society"—referring to decreasing birth rates and increasing life expectancies of adults and older people. Simultaneously, the socially shared conceptions of how to age well have changed dramatically over the last decades. An empirical analysis of public discourses about ageing over a period of 25 years reconstructs three story lines that give voices to distinct images of ageing: the "retirement," the "restless age," and the "productive age" narratives (Denninger, van Dyck, Lessenich, & Richter, 2014).

The core meaning of the classical term of retirement (*Ruhestand*) is that of an older person retiring, suggesting that he or she is legitimately liberated from work or relieved of any other (public) responsibility, and thus can enjoy the deserved eve of life, financed by public pension schemes. At the same time the term retirement depicts older people as "being tired" and disengaging from (any) social activities, which gives the idea of retirement a negative connotation as well—a proposition that was coined by structural functionalist theories of ageing in the 1960s (Klott, 2014).

Against this traditional understanding of retirement, a second story line and image of ageing has emerged in the late 1980s, i.e., the "rest-less age" (*Unruhestand*) mirroring the "active ageing" paradigm that began in the 1990s. Taking the image of the retired old person as a negative counterpart, this new notion (re-)constructs elderly people as "best agers" with the image of the well-off, open-minded, and cosmopolitan pensioner engaging in time-consuming leisure activities for the sake of individual fulfilment and self-realization. In the late 1990s a new narrative emerged, *productive ageing*, which has subsequently dominated the public discourse on old age and ageing in Germany. The general idea behind this new term and image is that older people could—and actually should—make use of their resources not only for themselves, but also for society, including grand-parenting, civic engagement, and community work. This new story line goes along with a recent pension reform in Germany, where the enforced retirement age will gradually rise from 56 to 67 up to the year 2031. Denninger et al. (2014) identify a sequence of these three story lines evolving one after the other, but nowadays they are mutually overlapping and interfering images of ageing, with a prominent focus on the active and productive ageing paradigm.

This public discourse about getting older in Germany reveals that today old age and ageing has a broad set of meanings for the elderly, who are expected to enjoy their deserved freedom, have time for leisure activities, actively engage in grand-parenting, engage in community work, or participate in traveling. Only a small minority unconditionally agrees with and lives up to this *productive ageing* image. Instead, retirement and old age is highly valued by most of our interviewees because of its freedom of self-determination. Denninger et al. (2014) even identify a majority of attitudes that challenge any popular "active ageing" narratives. Focusing on the dimension of physical activities in the active ageing paradigm, Hartmann-Tews, Tischer, and Combrink (2012) contrarily found a relevant proportion of elderly people engaging in physical activities as an important tool to stay fit and healthy in order to play an active role in society.

Parallel to the rise of the active ageing paradigm, researchers in the fields of sports sciences and sports medicine have addressed the functional decrements, normally associated with the ageing process, suggesting that certain exercise interventions can reduce or even prevent the functional declines linked to ageing in general. It seems that sport scientists and medical researchers all over the world have successfully positioned themselves as key players in the fight against ageing. Physical activity continues to be a key factor for the prevention and management of many risk factors and functional disabilities associated with ageing up to very old age (Paterson, Govindasamy, Vidmar, Cunningham, & Koval, 2004). The increasing evidences about the positive relationship between exercise and physical and cognitive functions has had its effects on society. The idea of promoting exercise as an instrument for individualized risk management has been endorsed by (neoliberal) government policies in many Western countries. But there are critical voices as well. In her critical review about the role of sport sciences within the anti-ageing discourse, Tulle rightly points out that "the (scientific) reconstruction of the ageing body as trainable and fit has an anti-ageing remit, in that it is geared toward the elimination of ageing as process and burden" (2008, 346).

Besides the sociological research on images of ageing and the role of sport science within this development there is a growing academic interest about the social framing of (in-)active lifestyles of elderly people. The following section presents data and evidence about the social structures of participation in sport and physical activities of older people.

Development of participation in sport and physical activity of the elderly

Older people are not a homogeneous group as often suggested; instead they are characterized by diversity with respect to educational level, professional status, income and means, health status, family ties, resources of time, and many more aspects. Despite this diversity, among the elderly population empirical studies reveal a trend and some patterns with respect to their participation in sports and physical activities.

There have been several surveys in Germany over the past 30 years that present data about the participation rate of older people in physical activity and sports. The main stock of surveys produces cross-sectional data, i.e., information on activities of different age groups at a certain point of time. All empirical studies document a negative relationship between age and participation in sports. Participation in sports is predominantly a leisure time activity of children and adolescents, and it systematically decreases across the age groups: Older people show lower participation rates than the younger ones. It is important to note that this finding does not describe the individual development during life, as a description of this kind can only be derived from longitudinal data, which will be addressed in the next section. The participation rates documented in the surveys for people aged 50+ vary between 30 percent and 60 percent (e.g., Becker et al., 2007; Deutsches Institut für Wirtschaftsforschung (DIW), 2015; Ellert, Wirtz, & Ziese, 2006; Hartmann-Tews, Tischer, & Combrink, 2012). Comparing the data of the various studies presents some methodological challenges.

First of all, the answers to the questions of participation rates in physical activities and sports vary from survey to survey as a result of the differing thematic cores of the surveys. In addition, the exact wording of the question about the participation in physical activities and sports and the given options to respond to the questions vary as well. Particularly striking is the fact that the participation rates reported in surveys that focus on health and sports are generally much higher than participation rates in surveys that cover more general themes, and in which sport is only a minor issue. In order to develop an answer to the question whether older people are part of the sportification process, there is only one survey to refer to, the German Socioeconomic Panel (SOEP). This survey has a twofold design as it is a regularly performed as a representative cross-sectional survey and a longitudinal survey as well. It focuses mainly on the socio-economic development with only a few questions on physical activity patterns (DIW, 2015).

According to this survey, regular participation in sport and physical activity for at least 1 hour a week has increased for all age groups over the last 30 years, and in particular for people 45+ in age: the increase in participation has been reported as 26 percentage points in the age group of 16–24 year olds and about 35 percentage points for those 45+ years of age. Social changes and the involved sportification of society obviously had stronger effects on adults and the elderly than it had on the younger age groups. This in turn leads to the finding that the general effects of ageing have become smaller over the past decades, meaning people are actively participating in slowing down their ageing process (Becker & Klein, 2007; Eichberg & Rott, 2004; Lampert, Mensink, & Ziese, 2005).

The academic literature on physical activity and participation in sports has often identified the so-called gender gap, i.e., the fact that fewer girls and women are regularly participating in physical activities and sport than boys and men. However, recent studies document a more heterogeneous picture of gender differences in general and specifically with respect to the elderly. While the SOEP data as well as some other studies show a significantly higher participation rate of women 50+ (DIW, 2015; Robert Koch Institut, 2009) other surveys do not and even present a higher proportion of men aged 50+ engaging in physical activity (Becker et al., 2007; Hinrichs et al., 2010). This diminishing or blurring of the traditional gender gap in participation is due to the fact that participation rates of girls and women in all age groups have increased significantly more than that of the boys and men (Becker & Schneider, 2005; Lampert, Mensink, & Ziese, 2005). Focusing on the development between 1985 and 2013, the socioeconomic panel identifies the strongest increase of participation by boys and men in the age groups 45+ with the single strongest increase in the age group 65–74 (34 percentage points from 12 percent to 46 percent). The strongest increase of participation of girls and women covers the same age groups 45+ with the strongest increase between the 65–74 years old (42 percentage points from 10 percent to 52 percent).

General population surveys unanimously indicate a correlation between social class, including social stratification, such as educational level, professional status, income/means, and participation in sports: The higher the social strata the higher the participation rate of people engaging in sport and physical activity (Rohrer & Haller, 2015). These findings are in accordance with participation profiles of elderly people, which signifies a strong correlation between social class and sport participation of the elderly (Becker et al., 2007; Hartmann-Tews, Tischer, & Combrink, 2012; Hinrichs et al., 2010). Most of the surveys produce cross-sectional data and inform about the amount of people who participate in physical activities at a defined point of time or period of time. Very few surveys pursue a longitudinal research design. SOEP is the only data set providing information about sport participation through long-term, non-retrospective methods since it is based on a sample of identical persons since 1984. In addition, the Interdisciplinary Longitudinal Study of Adult Development (ILSE) includes data about physical activities and sport participation of the elderly, based on a sample of two cohorts (years of birth 1930–1933 and 1950–1952) that were interviewed and tested physically in a 4-year interval (Eichberg & Rott, 2004).

In sum, the data documents two findings that seem to be contradictory. On the one hand, surveys indicate a high stability of participation in physical activities and sport profiles across the lifespan; and on the other hand, they document a high variation of participation throughout life. Continuity and stability in participation can be identified insofar as there is a majority of people who either show continuous and long-lasting sport participation or a long-lasting inactivity (Klein & Becker, 2008). At the same time, there are many patterns of discontinuous participation. This is the case when people stop their regular physical activities in youth and get back to being active at a later point in life or when sedentary adults become physically active only in advanced age (Eichberg & Rott, 2004). There is only one significant general feature, the amount of inactive people as a whole is continuously growing with advancing age, which is called the *age-effect* (Becker & Klein, 2007). The results of cross-sectional studies and longitudinal studies therefore complement each other in this finding.

The age-effect is significant even when the health status of elderly people is controlled (Erlinghagen, 2003). This finding is important as it refutes traditional stereotypes that decreasing participation in physical activities and sport is due to deteriorating health. It calls attention to a variety of other social circumstances that influence the decisions to stay or to become physically active or not, such as changing cultural values (ideal of fitness, individual responsibility of well-being, lifestyle elements), social norms (health insurance, pension schemes), and individual resources (time and money). Therefore, the tendency of an age-effect does not reflect an outstanding trend of an increasing disengagement of physical activity and sport across the course of life; it rather masks the diversity of discontinuous participation. Results from a qualitative retrospective study conducted with older people indicate that participation in physical activities and sport in early tend to increase the probability to be physically active on old age (Klostermann & Nagel, 2011).

With respect to the potential influence of socio-economic variables— such as income, educational level, and occupational status—on the development of participation over the life span only a minor stock of research is documented. On the basis of the data collected by ILSE, the authors identify education and income as important factors to influence continuity of sport while gender and age show no discriminating effect (Eichberg & Rott, 2004). Findings from a study with a retrospective research design support these results. Higher education levels correlate positively with continuous sports activity, and cultural capital seems to be more important than economic capital (Becker et al., 2007; Klein, 2009).

Sport selection by the elderly, motives, and preferred settings

Only few surveys gather information about preferred physical activities or sports and their respective settings. There seems to be a tendency of older people to adapt physical activities to declining physical fitness with advancing age. Whereas adults in their 30s and 40s prefer individual sports such as jogging and fitness sports, elderly prefer various ways of gymnastics, swimming, and functional training, and physical activities that can easily be integrated in daily life, such as (nordic) walking and cycling (Hartmann-Tews, Tischer, & Combrink, 2012; Thiel, Huy, & Gomolinsky, 2008). Gender-specific profiles with regard to preferred physical activities are visible across all age groups—alongside a huge and dominant amount of physical activities and sport of the elderly that indicate no significant differences in participation rates. Among the elderly, a gender profile is characterized by male preferences for jogging and cycling and female preferences of all kinds of gymnastics including aerobic and aqua-fitness (Hartmann-Tews, Tischer, & Combrink, 2012). This gender profile can partly be explained by culturally established gendered connotations of sports. There are still stereotypes about the gender adequacy of physical activities and sports that in turn represent a symbolic barrier for men to participate in "female" sports or for women to participate in "male" sports (Hartmann-Tews & Tischer, 2008). These stereotypes and connotations of sport activities represent a social framework that influences the decisions whether to take part in the existing offers of sport clubs and other institutions.

The preferred settings of physical activities of older people are informally organized activities without an institutional frame. Sports clubs rank second and commercial organizations rank third in the list of settings. There are significantly more men than women enrolled as members of a sports club but there is some evidence that older men remain members in sports clubs even when they are physically inactive and do not participate in training sessions (Hartmann-Tews, Tischer, & Combrink, 2012). In contrast, commercially run organizations and public offers are more often chosen by elderly women.

Findings on elderly people's attitudes toward sports and on motivations to participate in sport and physical activities are as heterogeneous as data on participation. This is due to varying research designs in general and different conceptualization of "attitudes," "motives," and "motivation" in particular. Two general findings can be summarized. First, cross-sectional data document a dominance of health-related motivation. Findings about the ranking of further components of motivation (i.e., social engagement, recreation, achievement) vary a lot and are sometimes even contradictory (Hartmann-Tews, Tischer, & Combrink, 2012; Thiel, Huy, & Gomolinsky, 2008). Second, it seems that older women and men have more or less the same attitudes toward physical activities. Various studies confirm that attitudes and motives focusing on the dimension of health and fun are unanimously shared by elderly people irrespective of their sex. However, two recent studies on health behavior and physical activities of the elderly add interesting gender-typical differentiation to the stock of knowledge. Older women aged 55–75 put significantly more emphasis on the "anti-ageing" functions of physical activity than elderly men, as they rate higher on items related to sports participation in order to prevent frailty, focusing on the training of flexibility, testing performance, and staying independent of outside care in the long term. In addition, and in contrast to traditional findings, older women agreed more on the motivation factor "experiencing achievements" than did older men (Hartmann-Tews, Tischer, & Combrink, 2008). With regard to health behavior and physical activity, older women are characterized more often as being "fit and performance hungry" rather than as being "conventional" and "easy going and committed" (Huy & Thiel, 2009).

Conclusion—staying physically active in times of active ageing

Older people are a prominent part of the so-called sportification in Germany, since the increase of participation in sports and physical activities over the past decades has been stronger with respect to the older people (aged 45+) than with youth and young cohorts. This increase in participation rates has been more prominent among women than men across all age groups. Against this backdrop the traditional gender gap in participation is diminishing or even reversing. However, all empirical cross-sectional studies document a correlation between age and participation in sports: the older the age group the lower the participation rates are, but the age gap has become closer.

When older people (65–85 years old) are asked what they think they can do to stay healthy and fit, the second most common answer is "to mind sufficient physical activity" (Generali Deutschland AG, 2017, 156). This statement corresponds to the knowledge conveyed by sports science and sport medicine and reflects the active ageing paradigm that has been successfully established over the past decades in Germany. Sociological studies indicate, that (older) people have understood the message. The cultural idea(l) of active ageing has become a broadly shared social expectation. Empirical data even show that physical activity and staying healthy up to old age is seen as an "individual duty and social responsibility" by some of the elderly (Hartmann-Tews, Tischer, & Combrink, 2012, 86). Although the cultural idea(l) of active ageing is widely shared, the adoption of this image and a physically active lifestyle is socially stratified. Significantly fewer elderly individuals from lower socio-economic classes support the notion that there is a need for sufficient physical exercise to stay healthy and fit in old age, and correspondingly fewer of them are physically active (Generali Deutschland AG, 2017). Therefore it may well be that the active ageing paradigm is mirrored by the "new elderly" in particular, the post-war cohorts of the wealthy, healthy, and educated "young elderly" currently *moving* into retirement.

References

Becker, S. & Klein, T. (2007). Altern und Sport—zur Veränderung der sportlichen Aktivität im Lebenslauf. In H.W. Wahl & H. Mollenkopf (Eds.), *Alternsforschung am Beginn des 21. Jahrhunderts* (pp. 287–305). Berlin: AKA.

Becker, S. & Schneider, S. (2005). Analysen zur Sportbeteiligung auf der Basis des repräsentativen Bundes-Gesundheitssurveys 1998. *Sport und Gesellschaft, 2(2),* 173–204.

Becker, S., Huy, C., Brinkhoff, K.-P., Gomolinsky, U., Klein, T., Thiel, A., & Zimmermann-Stenzel, M. (2007). Ein aktives Leben leben—Sport, Bewegung und Gesundheit im mittleren und höheren Erwachsenenalter. Konzeption, Datenerhebung und erste Ergebnisse eines repräsentativen Basis-Survey für die 50–70-jährige baden-württembergische Wohnbevölkerung. *Gesundheitswesen,* 69, 401–407.

Denninger, T., van Dyck, S., Lessenich, S., & Richter, A. (2014). *Leben im Ruhestand. Zur Neuverhandlung des Alters in der Aktivgesellschaft.* Bielefeld: Transcript.

Deutsches Institut für Wirtschaftsforschung Berlin (2015). *Das Sozioökonomische Panel. Instrumente und Feldarbeit.* Retrieved from www.diw.de/deutsch.

Eichberg, S. & Rott, C. (2004). Sportverhalten im mittleren und höheren Erwachsenenalter. Bedingungsfaktoren für Kontinuität und Diskontinuität. *Journal of Public Health 12(2),* 93–104.

Ellert, U., Wirtz, J., & Ziese, T. (2006). *Telefonischer Gesundheitssurvey des Robert-Koch-Instituts (2. Welle). Beiträge zur Gesundheitsberichterstattung des Bundes.* Berlin: RKI.

Erlinghagen, M. (2003). *Wer treibt Sport im geteilten Deutschland? Graue Reihe des Instituts Arbeit und Technik 2003–04.* Retrieved from www.iatge.de/aktuell/veroeff/2003/gr2003-04.pdf.

Generali Deutschland AG (2017). *Generali Altersstudie 2017. Wie ältere Menschen in Deutschland denken und leben.* Berlin: Springer.

Hartmann-Tews, I. (1998). *Sport für alle!? Strukturwandel europäischer Sportsysteme im Vergleich.* Schorndorf: Hofmann.

Hartmann-Tews, I. (2017). *Senior_innen in Bewegung—Beobachtungen zur Relevanz von Geschlecht und Alter in verschiedenen Sport-Settings.* In G. Sobiech & S. Günther (Eds.), *Sport & Gender. (Inter-)nationale sportsoziologische Geschlechterforschung: Theoretische Ansätze, Praktiken und Perspektiven* (pp. 235–251). Wiesbaden: Springer VS.

Hartmann Tews, I. & Tischer, U. (2008). Alter(n) und sportliche Aktivität—auf den Spuren sozialer Deutungsmuster im höheren Lebensalter. *Spectrum der Sportwissenschaften, 2(2),* 39–58.

Hartmann-Tews, I., Tischer, U., & Combrink, C. (2008). Doing Gender und Doing Age im Kontext von Sport und Bewegung. *Zeitschrift für Frauenforschung & Geschlechterstudien, 2(2),* 32–51.

Hartmann-Tews, I., Tischer, U., & Combrink, C. (2012). *Bewegtes Alter(n)— Sozialstrukturelle Analysen von Sport im Alter.* Leverkusen: Barbara Budrich.

Hinrichs, T., Trampisch, U., Burghaus, I., Endres, H.G., Klaaßen-Mielke, R., Moschny, A., & Platen, P. (2010). Correlates of sport participation among community-dwelling elderly people in Germany: a cross-sectional study. *European Review of Aging and Physical Activity, 7(2),* 105–115.

Huy, C. & Thiel, A. (2009). Altersbilder und Gesundheitsverhalten. Theorie und empirischer Befund zum Einfluss individueller Vorstellungen vom Alter(n) auf das Gesundheitsverhalten. *Zeitschrift für Gesundheitspsychologie, 17(3),* 121–132.

Klein, T. (2009). Determinanten der Sportaktivität und der Sportart im Lebenslauf. *Kölner Zeitschrift für Soziologie und Sozialpsychologie, 61,* 1–32.

Klein, T. & Becker, S. (2008). Gibt es wirklich eine Reduzierung sportlicher Aktivität im Lebenslauf? Eine Analyse alters- und kohortenbezogener Unterschiede der Sportaktivität. *Zeitschrift für Soziologie, 37(3),* 226–245.

Klostermann, C. & Nagel, S. (2011). Sport treiben ein Leben lang? *Sportwissenschaft, 41(3),* 216–232.

Klott, S. (2014). Theorien des Alters und des Alterns. In S. Becker & H. Brandenburg (Eds.), *Lehrbuch Gerontologie* (pp. 37–74). Bern: Huber.

Lampert, T., Mensink, G.B.M., & Ziese, T. (2005). Sport und Gesundheit bei Erwachsenen in Deutschland. *Bundesgesundheitsblatt—Gesundheitsforsch—Gesundheitsschutz 2005,* 1357–1364.

Paterson, D.H., Govindasamy, D., Vidmar, M., Cunningham, D.A., & Koval, J.J. (2004). Longitudinal study of determinants of dependence in an elderly population. *Journal of the American Geriatrics Society, 52,* 1632–1638.

Robert Koch-Institut (2009). *GEDA—Gesundheit in Deutschland aktuell.* Berlin: Oktoberdruck AG.

Rohrer, T. & Haller, M. (2015). Sport und soziale Ungleichheit—Neue Befunde aus dem internationalen Vergleich. *Kölner Zeitschrift für Soziologie und Sozialpsychologie, 67,* 57–82.

Thiel, A., Huy, C., & Gomolinsky, U. (2008). Alterssport in Baden-Wüttemberg—Präferenzen, Motive und Settings für die Sportaktivität in der Generation 50+. *Deutsche Zeitschrift für Sportmedizin, 59(7–8)*, 163–167.

Tulle, E. (2008). Acting your age? Sports science and the ageing body. *Journal of Aging Studies, 22*, 340–347.

Chapter 3

Global aging in Portugal

Pedro G. Carvalho, Ana Pereira,
Anabela Almeida, Rita Palmeira-de-Oliveira,
and Aldo M. Costa

Introduction

In 1948, the World Health Organization (WHO) defined health as "a state of complete physical, mental and social well-being and not only the absence of disease" (World Health Organization, 1948, 2006, 1). Three large dimensions in a context of illness were considered: physical, mental, and social. In the 1960s, driven by economic development, after the end of World War II, the concept of "quality of life" began to be introduced in political discourses (Pimentel, 2006).

The world trends in human life activity highlight that health is beyond a physician, a hospital, or an illness problem. Feeling healthy also affects productivity; therefore, it is very important to fully understand human well-being, the physical and mental personality, and consequently policies. In health policy, the term "diagnosis" is not always suitable, and this will sometimes open incentives for wrong policy responses (Carvalho, 2016). The world population is experiencing an aging process together with a decrease in new birth rates and fertility in western societies, along with an increase in the life expectancy rate. The 1960s also brought about women's emancipation to search for jobs and diminish the willingness to have lots of kids and large families. Grandparents in Portugal play an important role taking care of kids while both members of the couples are going to work. Additionally, we observe an inversion between youth and elderly percentages, which impairs the world demographic renovation capacity and increases the dependency rate. Therefore, lowering the number of contributors paying for health and insurance systems will raise the volume of financial needs to keep a healthy imbalance across generations. According to the European Commission (European Commission, 2009), age pyramids are becoming larger on the top; in 2010, it was estimated we have 524 million individuals over 65 years of age (8 percent of the world population); moreover, this number is expected to rise to over 1.5 billion individuals in 2050 (doubling to 16 percent of the world population).

Considering the less developed countries in the 2050 horizon, the EU predicted the aging population would increase by 250 percent, resulting in the life expectancy rate increasing to 0.2 percent and 0.7 percent in Asia and Europe, respectively (Carrilho & Gonçalves, 2004; European Commission, 2009). From the beginning of the twentieth until the beginning of the twenty-first century, life expectancy went from 50 to 80 years!

In Portugal, life expectancy is 78 years for men and 83 years for women (European Commission, 2009), although 60 years is the expected healthy period for the elderly, which points to tough measures being required to improve the quality of life. There is little joy, however, in living longer if the quality of functional and emotional life is poor. More recently, Census data (INE, 2012) revealed that approximately 12 percent of the resident population and 60 percent (400,964 individuals) of the elderly live alone or in the exclusive company of other older people (804,577 individuals). This is a new phenomenon, the dimension of which has increased by nearly 28 percent after 2000. Traditionally, the elderly used to continue living with their families after retirement. With democracy, in 1974, Portugal created a National Health System that improved health care for its citizens, thereby increasing life expectancy for its people.

The healthy life expectancy of 65 years of age is 9.9 years for men and 9.0 for women (Saúde, 2015), which follows the EU pattern of aging (13.9 and 15.2 in Sweden and on EU average, 12.9 and 11.7). The increase in life expectancy relates to scientific progress of diagnostic and treatment resources for a wide variety of diseases associated with aging. Chronic diseases are quite prevalent among the older population and multi-morbidity (defined as more than two concomitant diseases) is related to disability in this population (Rizzuto, Melis, Angleman, Qiu, & Marengoni, 2017). Hypertension is present in more than 60 percent of those aged above 65 and is considered a risk factor for vascular cerebral accident, myocardia (Mostofsky, Penner, & Mittleman, 2014) and peripheral vascular complications (Ebrahim, Taylor, Ward, Beswick, Burke, Davey, & Smith, 2011). Consequently, they require careful diagnosis and treatments prescribed in prevention protocols (Ruivo & Alcântara, 2012).

Depending upon the associated risk factors, such as age, gender, and degenerative processes, prevention is crucial to avoid the emergence of other related pathologies (such as sleep apnea), endocrine diseases (e.g., diabetes, obesity) and psychiatric disorders (e.g., psychosis) (Evans, Wang, & Morris, 2002; Gonzaga, Bertolami, Bertolami, Amodeo, & Calhounet, 2015; Vancampfort et al., 2015). Rheumatoid arthritis and osteoporosis are often associated with elderly lifestyles (e.g., level and type of physical exercise), affecting regions of the body (elbow, knee, hip, spine) that condition functional independence and quality of life (Hiligsmann, Cooper, Arden, Boers, Branco, Luisa Brandi, & Bruyère, 2013). In addition, malnutrition associated with digestive diseases and degeneration of tissues and organs may favor the development of other diseases such as urinary incontinence or the fragility of pelvic floor muscles (Rubenstein, Harker, Salva, Guigoz, & Vellas, 2001). Neurological diseases (Alzheimer's and Parkinson's diseases) are also frequent in the elderly and are associated with loss of function and quality of life, especially daily tasks. It is well established that neuronal structures decline with age, indicated by a decrease in memory capacity, attention, decision making, comprehension, speech, and psychomotor functions (Small, Dixon, McArdle, & Grimm, 2012). These changes have implications in day-to-day life, as they cause a penchant for falling risk, learning time, and decision-making ability.

Another aspect of multi-morbidity is the intrinsic relation with drug prescription that leads to polypharmacy (generally defined as the concurrent use of several drugs), which represents a major public health problem by itself (Strehblow, Smeikal, & Fasching, 2014; Wyles & Rehman, 2005). In fact, it has been suggested that the theoretical probability of drug-to-drug interactions (that can result in adverse drug reactions) is up to 50 percent when a patient is taking five different drugs and reaches 100 percent for seven concomitant drugs (Delafuente, 2003). These adverse drug reactions are often misinterpreted as symptoms of new medical conditions leading to the prescription of more drugs representing the so-called "prescribing cascade" (Rochon & Gurwitz, 2017).

It is important, however, to consider that not all elderly adults are affected by serious health problems and decline of cognitive function. In fact, there are investigations that demonstrate that some centenarian individuals do not present any alteration of cognitive function, which also reflects the plasticity capacity of the neural network that can be stimulated with diversified experiences.

Participation in physical activity and exercise can diminish cognitive decline, contributing to the reduction of the risk of dementia, control of cognitive performance, health, and depression. The practice of regular exercise seems to have a protective effect on nerve cells, promoting neurogenesis and, in addition, genes that interfere in the structure and adaptability of synapses affected by physical exercise. In other words, as we age, having an active and socially diverse lifestyle is at the core of preventing declines and optimizing psychomotor functioning. Exercise plays a fundamental role because it is a strategic factor and is focused specifically on different levels of prevention (Laforge, Rossi, Prochaska, Velicer, Levesque, & McHorney, 1999).

With the change in values over the last two decades, social and psychological needs of older people are given more attention. Researchers in the economic and social sciences of western societies have focused on determining the indicators for establishing and measuring the well-being of populations (Jonker, Gerritsen, Bosboom, & Van Der Steen, 2004), including mortality, morbidity, per capita income, level of employment, and formal education (Pimentel, 2006).

Quality of life

Measuring Health Related Quality of Life (HRQoL) is a valid indicator for health systems evaluation and has been heavily valued in the last decades (Alonso, Ferrer, Gandek, Ware, & Aaronson, 2004; Antonelli-Incalzi, Pedone, Scarlata, Battaglia, & Scichilone, 2009; Franzen, Blomqvist, & Saveman, 2006; Lefante Jr., Harmon, Ashby, Barnard, & Webber, 2005; Johansson, Dahiström, & Broström, 2006; Jensen, Saunders, Thierer, & Friedman, 2008; Moffatt & Mackintosh, 2009; Patrick & Erickson, 1993; Revicki, 1993; Romero et al., 2013; Van der Waal, Terwee, Van der Windt, Bouter, & Dekker, 2005; Wagner et al., 2008). Depending upon the need to know if certain health interventions have made differences, several HRQoL measurement systems have been developed.

Considering the rising costs and the inability of the health system to provide full coverage of the demand for services, these systems have been increasingly applied in the allocation of resources and in the selection of interventions to be implemented (Hays, Anderson, & Revicki, 2000). Thus, the use of HRQoL measures has been of interest to professionals to monitor the results of interventions. Attention has been drawn to health sector managers to consider the health status of the population and the selection of technologies, including mechanisms of organization of the health system that can more effectively promote the current health profile (Hays, Anderson, & Revicki, 2000; Revicki, 1993). Techniques for measuring health status and HRQoL provide information regarding the benefits and risks of medical treatment, taking into account the perspective of physicians, patients, and society.

Consequently, the importance of systems of cultural significance and the meaning of life quality goes far beyond symptomatology and the effects of disease in an individual's functional state. The impact of the disease must be assessed according to traditional medical measures, remembering its influence on the individual's quality of life (Pibernik-Okanović, 2001). Individual expectations vary, especially as a result of the effect of the therapy and their well-being relative to the disease. Thus, it is important to evaluate each person's perception of health status and expectations regarding treatment (Pimentel, 2006; Santos, Almedia, & Rosado, 2016).

In a society where average life expectancy is increasing, coupled with an increase in the number of elderly, it is of utmost importance to know the aging cycle, how people age, and who cares for them in the final stage of life. In summary, Schwartzmann (2007) justifies the need to use HRQoL measures because:

1   Decision making in the health sector should take into account user perceptions supported by scientific knowledge that considers classical quantitative indicators (morbidity, life expectancy), costs, and

qualitative indicators that express the impact of quality of life (life and patient satisfaction).

2   Analysis of the health care process should be performed in terms of technical assessment and interpersonal excellence.

3   The study of the factors that determine the patient's perception in different moments of life and of the diseases that interfere in the health-related quality of life allow to recognize the mechanisms that influence it.

4   Exclusively cost-based decisions are unacceptable from an ethical point of view.

Scientific knowledge and best practices

Anti-aging strategies must be developed based upon the biological mechanisms underlying functional decline. Although the aging process is multifactorial and complex (Fonseca, 2005), there is a set of theories: *stochastic*—based on environmental changes that lead to successive lesions, and *deterministic*—based on genotypic characteristics, that support and complement this phenomenon (Cristofalo, 1988). Individual aging, however, is determined by genetic and environmental factors, both capable of altering gene expression and the aging phenotype. Certain cellular and molecular changes that contribute more significantly than others include telomere shortening, epigenetic changes and loss of protein homeostasis, metabolic dysregulation due to chronic adaptation to injury, mitochondrial dysfunction and cellular senescence, and regenerative tissue decline and inflammatory response (Maguire & Slater, 2013).

Therefore, when we talk about the decline in cellular functionality associated with aging, the aim has often been to focus on the changes associated with mitochondria, because promising strategies for active and healthy aging are aimed at the maintenance of *sirtuin-mediated proteostasis*, as well as the practice of moderate and regular exercise (Gundersen, 2011; Martins, 2007). The solutions that aim to improve the quality of life in the elderly require a comprehensive scientific knowledge, especially about the morphological, biological, and social processes that affect aging. Strategic guidelines, community projects, and good practices in this area should value human dignity, active and independent living, and intergenerational relations, thereby contributing to valuing the economy of old age. This is a multidisciplinary task requiring much from different health care professionals who must discuss and prescribe appropriately.

The WHO has launched *Move for Health*, an annual global initiative to promote physical activity as a key factor for health and well-being of the general population. This has had repercussions in the development of effective intervention strategies and research projects in Portugal, namely in the increasing involvement of academic research units with community approach. The implementation of these programs seems to be associated also with the pressure to reduce costs related to health care by around 3.4 million euros (Laureano, Martins, Sousa, Machado-Rodrigues, Valente-Santos, & Coelho-e-Silva, 2014), taking the example of the National Programme for the Promotion of Physical and Sports Activity-Moves ("Mexe-te") (Instituto do Desporto de Portugal, 2004).

There are significant differences between the desired levels of physical activity. Researchers have shown that the most active elderly women presented the highest means in the physical and psychological domains. Additionally, sedentary individuals, when compared to active individuals, were less likely to present high levels of quality of life (Toscano & Oliveira, 2009). The actions directed toward physical activity are not intended merely to occupy the free time of the elderly or treat them as incapable individuals. Rather, programs should be preceded by information on the benefits of the regular engagement in physical activities, assessment of specific conditions, needs and expectations of this part of the population, in relation to achieve behavioral changes (Toscano & Oliveira, 2009). One of the most neglected issues is the layout and attendance in special academies or gyms that comfortably accommodate elderly people.

Programs in Portugal

In Portugal, the European Innovation Partnership on Active and Healthy Aging and the *Porto4Aging* consortium (around 80 institutions) have actively contributed to the operationalization of an innovative model based on a framework that favors joint networking. The partnership is composed of policy makers and health care providers, universities and research centers, business and industry, and civil society. All *Porto4Aging* partners are involved with various local, regional, national, or international initiatives, revitalized around the idea of active and healthy aging processes. This Centre for Excellence in Active and Healthy Aging in Porto has developed several interesting projects, namely:

- *Centenarios*—a photographic project that portrays the centennial population of the metropolitan area of Porto.
- *Adding Quality to Life—ADD LIFE*—an intergenerational learning with grandparents and grandchildren.
- *Well Aging III*—promoting the quality of life of elderly, physical, mental, and social well-being by encouraging active aging.
- *Bone Biochemical and Biomechanic Integrated Modeling*—focusing on bone remodeling processes and diseases, with the goal of developing novel models that integrate knowledge from bone physiology and its biochemical environment, biomechanics and geometric regulations, among others.

Aging@Coimbra is also a program seeking to create, develop, and implement good practices that contribute to the challenges posed by an aging society. The aim is to stimulate good practices that lead to an increase in the life span of citizens, giving them more years to live. Good practices contribute to raising the quality of life of citizens during the aging process. Some examples are:

- *Pantufinhas*—an electric bus that transports elderly people in an urban environment with accessibility difficulties.
- *Move*—an electric car, without a driver, that allows the horizontal transport of citizens having difficulty of movement.
- *Physiosensing*—a platform to monitor physical exercise.
- *Giraffplus*—a robot that accompanies elderly people who live alone and monitors their health parameters.

Furthermore, the Institute of Education and Citizenship plays an active role in the dissemination of science in rural areas and among others, e.g., *Life Stories*, a program that inspires through real life stories of an active and healthy lifestyle.

Considering the impact that multi-morbidity and polypharmacy in older adults have on the quality of life and physical activity, it is expected that a greater interest will be devoted to this topic. Recently, a project designed to improve the therapeutic management of the elderly (*Medicar Melhor*) commenced in a hospital located at the inner center region of Portugal (Centro Hospitalar Cova da Beira, Covilhã). This project aims to improve everyday clinical practice by raising awareness on the most frequent "potentially inappropriate medications" prescribed for the elderly and on the recommended best practices for therapeutic prescription (and "deprescribing") for this population.

The Institute of Aging (Instituto do Envelhecimento) at the University of Lisbon is a research unit focusing on the interdisciplinary investigations of aging (sociology, psychology, anthropology, economics, law, geography) with links to Biomedicine and Epidemiology. In recent years some innovative programs have been developed in Portugal, such as the introduction of innovative elements in everyday life of the elderly, suggestions of practices for active aging rather than merely aging physically, and more. Examples of these programs include the Senior University and Senior Tourism. The Senior Universities have contributed to improving the quality of life and value of the elderly (around 50,000 people), through active participation in different areas, including technology, arts, languages, and dance, as well as intellectual and cultural activities as a service to the community. Senior Tourism is also under development because Portugal presents favorable facilities providing adequate services for the elderly, such as thermal spas, outdoor itineraries, and culturally diversified sight-seeing. Social innovation and active aging promote entrepreneurship as a support for a knowledge-based society as the basis of the Europe 2020 strategy.

Considering the concept, we have developed above (HRQoL) the great challenges faced by an aging society require bold and powerful solutions with great impact. The European Commission, through the European Partnership for Active and Healthy Aging, fosters the need to create space for innovation based on knowledge and technology to generate new solutions. In Portugal, we are experiencing a great push for programs that help to build cities that are friendly to functionality needed by the elderly. This is a priority in the actions of the WHO—open spaces and buildings policy; transport; housing; participation, respect and social inclusion; civic participation and employment; communication and information; and community support and health service are some of the main examples and best practices.

Relationship between physical activity and health

The importance of understanding physical activity as a major component in the overall health of the elderly is stressed in recent investigations conducted on the overmedication many older people are receiving. Research performed in Portuguese community pharmacies found that the mean number of drugs taken by older adults was 7.3; 50 percent took six to nine drugs daily (CEFAR, 2009). These data are in accordance with international findings concerning polypharmacy, which is known to negatively influence health outcomes and quality of life (Delafuente, 2003; Montiel-Luque, Nunez-Montenegro, Martin-Aurioles, Canca-Sanchez, Toro-Toro, Gonzalez-Correa, & Polipresact Research, 2017; Novaes, da Cruz, Lucchetti, Leite, & Lucchetti, 2017; Wyles & Rehman, 2005). It is also known that this population is at higher risk of presenting adverse drug reactions because of physiological, metabolic, and functional changes related to aging that influence both the effect of drugs (*pharmacodynamics*) and their physiologic pathways, from absorption to excretion (*pharmacokinetics*) (Midlöv, 2013). The knowledge that older patients should not be treated under the same guidelines as younger adults has led to the identification of potentially inappropriate medications (PIM) for the elderly, a concept related to drugs that should be avoided in this population either because they are not effective or because their risks outweigh their benefits, such as those that increase the risk of falls or those which may depress the central nervous system (Corsonello, Pranno, Garasto, Fabietti, Bustacchini, & Lattanzio, 2009).

Furthermore, to understand the relationship between the benefits of exercise and aging, it is important to analyze the type of stimulus in the orientation of physical exercise prescription that should be understood in a functional perspective. Thus, here we want to stress that aerobic endurance training can contribute to the maintenance and improvement of cardiovascular and cognitive function contributing to increased life expectancy (Ploughman, McCarthy, Bosse, Sullivan, & Corbett, 2008). Strength training can combat the decrease of muscle mass associated with sarcopenia and functional weakness (Pereira, Izquierdo, Silva, Costa, Bastos, Gonzalez-Badillo, & Marques, 2012). These adaptations will emerge in a set of additional benefits, from fall prevention, flexibility, and wellness, among others.

In addition to the above stated factors that characterize and influence the functional and social dependence of the elderly (including fragility, disability, chronic diseases, and polymedication, see: Fernández-Ballesteros, Robine, Walker, & Kalache, 2012; Pereira, Izquierdo, Silva, Costa, Bastos, Gonzalez-Badillo, & Marques, 2012; Sousa, Pires, Conceição, Nascimento, Grenha, & Braz, 2011), we must consider other problems such as social isolation and institutionalization. Both factors are associated with reduced economic capabilities and contribute significantly to the reduction of quality of life. In fact, the implications for public health are evident (DGS, 2004), and affect all societies in general, whether they are more and less developed (Fontaine, 2000). It is therefore essential to develop strategies to reconcile formal and informal support for the elderly, together with reforms and incentives, particularly with regard to the extension of working life (WHO, 2002) and promotion of healthy lifestyles (American Pyschological Association (APA), 2008). This challenge for contemporary societies is complex, multidimensional, and dependent on geographic and cultural specificities. The difficulty for an adequate response includes the speed of the inversion of the demographic, familial, economic, social, and psychological paradigms, as well as the change in family structure.

It is important to consider the elderly's perceptions of their own goals and concerns in relation to cultural and social contexts in which they live (Paúl, Fonseca, Martin, & Amado, 2005), as old age can also be a time of discovery, opportunities, and personal growth. The initiatives should aim at the development of an accepting environment and an adequate framework of motivation and learning, of responsibility and autonomy, avoiding reductionism and ageist attitudes (Bytheway, 2005; WHOQOL Group, 1995). It is important to coordinate interdisciplinary intervention efforts to promote the well-being of the elderly (Simões, 2005) and their full inclusion in society.

Conclusion

This chapter focuses on global aging by analyzing the major social transformations after World War II in Europe and its effects on Portugal, including the 1960s movement of women's emancipation as well as the subsequent changes of the traditional roles in families. Additionally, Portugal experienced the democratization in the midst of the 1970s when the National Health System was created, which proved to be an excellent mechanism to increase life expectancy. Unfortunately, it also contributed to an increase in drug medicine intake, which dramatically raised the costs in the system. Over the past decades as well, obesity, cardiovascular diseases, Type 2 diabetes, and other kinds of illnesses have increased at an unprecedented rate, demanding quick responses from the government and several public institutions. The active role that physical activity and sport can play in the prevention or slowing down of the development of these diseases that go along with aging becomes apparent for Portugal.

The need for multidisciplinary approaches to prevent and promote health for people of all ages has emerged, especially because society is aware of the burden everyone must bear by taking care of older people who deserve to live quality and dignified lives.

It is, however, important to discuss and alert the population that physical exercise must be supported by scientific research, and knowledge has to be updated regularly and related to the personal contexts and social conditions people live in. The description of a number of important programs that are in practice in the main cities of Portugal can serve as examples to spread this trend. These can be transformed into physical activity and social policies by decision makers.

References

Alonso, J., Ferrer, M., Gandek, B., Ware Jr., J.E., & Aaronson, N.K. (2004). Health-related quality of life associated with chronic conditions in eight countries: results from the International Quality of Life Assessment (IQOLA) Project. *Quality of Life Research 13*, 83–298.

American Psychological Association (APA) (2008). *Blueprint for change: achieving integrated health care for an aging population.* Washington, DC: American Psychological Association.

Antonelli-Incalzi, R., Pedone, C., Scarlata, S., Battaglia, S., & Scichilone, N. (2009). Correlates of mortality in elderly COPD patients: focus on health-related quality of life. *Respirology, 14*, 98–104.

Bytheway, B. (2005). Ageism. In M. Johnson, V. Bengtson, P. Coleman, & T. Kikwood (Eds.). *The Cambridge handbook of age and aging* (pp. 338–345). Cambridge: Cambridge University Press.

Carrilho, M.J. & Gonçalves, C. (2004). Dinâmicas territoriais do envelhecimento: análise exploratória dos resultados dos censos 91 e 2001. *Revista Estudos Demográficos, 36*, 175–191.

Carvalho, P.G. (2016). Health policies require new multidisciplinary approaches. *Hygiea Internationalis, 12*(1), 103–111.

CEFAR. (2009). Analisando o saco de medicamentos dos idosos. *Farmácia Observatório. Associação Nacional das Farmácias, 23*, 5.

Corsonello, A., Pranno, L., Garasto, S., Fabietti, P., Bustacchini, S., & Lattanzio, F. (2009). Potentially inappropriate medication in elderly hospitalized patients. *Drugs & Aging, 26*(1), 31–39.

Cristofalo, V.J. (1988). An overview of the theories of biological aging. In: J.E. Biren & V.L. Bergsten (Eds.). *Emergent theories of aging* (pp. 188–182). New York: Springer.

Delafuente, J.C. (2003). Understanding and preventing drug interactions in elderly patients. *Critical Reviews in Oncology/Hematology, 48*(2), 133–143.

DGS (2004). *Programmea Nacional para a Saúde das Pessoas Idosas.* Lisboa: Ministérios da Saúde.

DGS (2015). *Plano Nacional de Saúde—Revisão e Extensão a 2020.* Direção Geral de Saúde, Ministério da Saúde, Lisboa.

Ebrahim, S., Taylor, F., Ward, K., Beswick, A., Burke, M., Davey, & Smith, G. (2011). Multiple risk factor interventions for primary prevention of coronary heart disease. *Cochrane Database Systematic Reviews,* 1, CD001561.

European Commission (2009). *Ageing report: economic and budgetary projections for the EU-27 Member States (2008–2060).* Brussels: European Communities.

Evans, J.M., Wang, J., & Morris, A.D. (2002). Comparison of cardiovascular risk between patients with type 2 diabetes and those who had had a myocardial infarction: cross sectional and cohort studies. *British Medical Journal, 324,* 939–942.

Fernández-Ballesteros, R., Robine, J.M., Walker, A., & Kalache, A. (2012). Active aging: a global goal. *Current Gerontology and Geriatrics Research Volume 2013,* http://dx.doi.org/10.1155/2013/298012.

Fonseca, A.M. (2005). *Desenvolvimento humano e envelhecimento.* Lisboa: Climpsi Editores.

Fontaine, R. (2000). O Envelhecimento e as suas causas. In Fontaine, R. (org.), *Psicologia do Envelhecimento* (pp. 19–32). Lisboa: Climepsi Editores.

Franzen, K., Blomqvist, K., & Saveman, B.I. (2006). Impact of chronic heart failure on elderly persons' daily life: a validation study. *European Journal of Cardiovascular Nursing, 5,* 137–145.

Gonzaga, C., Bertolami, A., Bertolami, M., Amodeo, C., & Calhoun, D. (2015). Obstructive sleep apnea, hypertension and cardiovascular diseases. *Journal of Human Hypertension, 29,* 705–712.

Gundersen, K. (2011). Excitation-transcription coupling in skeletal muscle: the molecular pathways of exercise. *Biological Reviews of the Cambridge Philosophical Society, 86,* 564–600.

Hays, R.D., Anderson, R.T., & Revicki, D. (2000). Assessing reliability and validity of measurement in clinical trials. In M.J. Staquet, R.D. Hays, & P.M. Fayers (Eds.). *Quality of life assessment in clinical trials* (pp. 169–182). New York: Oxford University Press.

Hiligsmann, M., Cooper, C., Arden, N., Boers, M., Branco, J.C., Luisa Brandi, M., & Bruyère, O. (2013). Health economics in the field of osteoarthritis: an expert's consensus paper from the European Society for Clinical and Economic Aspects of Osteoporosis and Osteoarthritis (ESCEO) *Seminars in Arthritis and Rheumatism, 43,* 303–313.

Instituto do Desporto de Portugal (2004). A actividade física—O instrumento mais barato de saúde pública. In *Mexa-se*—Programmea Nacional de Promoção da Atividade Física e Desportiva (pp. 3–4). Lisboa.

Instituto Nacional de Estatística (2009). Projeções da População Residente em Portugal, 2008–2060, Lisboa.

Instituto Nacional de Estatística (2012). *Censos 2011*. Portugal, INE.

Jensen, P.M., Saunders, R.L., Thierer, T., & Friedman, B. (2008). Factors associated with oral health-related quality of life in community-dwelling elderly persons with disabilities. *Journal of the American Geriatric Society, 56*, 711–717.

Johansson, P., Dahiström, U., & Broström, A. (2006). Factors and interventions influencing health-related quality of life in patients with heart failure: a review of the literature. *European Journal of Cardiovascular Nursing, 5*, 5–15.

Jonker, C., Gerritsen, D.L., Bosboom, P.R., & Van Der Steen, J.T. (2004). A model for quality of life measures in patients with dementia: Lawton's next step. *Dementia and Geriatric Cognitive Disorders.* http://doi.org/10.1159/000079196.

Laforge, R.G., Rossi, J.S., Prochaska, J.O., Velicer, W.F., Levesque, D.A., & McHorney, C.A. (1999). *Stage of regular exercise and health-related quality of life, 28*, 349–360.

Laureano, M.L.M., Martins, R.A., Sousa, N.M., Machado-Rodrigues, A.M., Valente-Santos, J., & Coelho-e-Silva, M.J. (2014). Relationship between functional fitness, medication costs and mood in elderly people. *Revista da Associação Médica Brasileira, 60*, 200–207.

Lefante, Jr. J., Harmon, G.N., Ashby, K.M., Barnard, D., & Webber, L.S. (2005). Use of the SF-8 to assess health-related quality of life for a chronically ill, low-income population participating in the Central Louisiana Medication Access Programme (CMAP). *Quality of Life Research, 14*, 665–673.

Maguire, S.L., & Slater, B.M.J. (2013). Physiology of ageing. *Anaesthesia, Intensive Care Medicine, 14*, 310–312.

Martins, R. (2007). Envelhecimento, retrogénese do desenvolvimento motor, exercício físico e promoção da saúde. *Boletim da Sociedade Portuguesa de Educação Física, 32*, 31–40.

Midlöv, P. (2013). Pharmacokinetics and pharmacodynamics in the elderly. *OA Elderly Medicine, 1*(1), 1–5.

Moffatt, S. & Mackintosh, J. (2009). Older people's experience of proactive welfare rights advice: qualitative study of a South Asian community. *Ethnicity & Health, 14*, 5–25.

Montiel-Luque, A., Nunez-Montenegro, A.J., Martin-Aurioles, E., Canca-Sanchez, J. C., Toro-Toro, M.C., Gonzalez-Correa, J.A., & Polipresact Research, G. (2017). Medication-related factors associated with health-related quality of life in patients older than 65 years with polypharmacy. *PLoS One, 12*(2), e0171320. doi: 10.1371/journal.pone.0171320.

Mostofsky, E., Penner, E.A., & Mittleman, M.A. (2014). Outbursts of anger as a trigger of acute cardiovascular events: a systematic review and meta-analysis. *European Heart Journal, 35*, 1404–1410.

Novaes, P.H., da Cruz, D.T., Lucchetti, A.L.G., Leite, I.C.G., & Lucchetti, G. (2017). The "iatrogenic triad": polypharmacy, drug-drug interactions, and potentially inappropriate medications in older adults. *International Journal of Clinical Pharmacology.* doi: 10.1007/s11096-017-0470-2.

Patrick, D.L. & Erickson, P. (1993). Concepts of health-related quality of life. In C.J.L. (Ed.). *Designing and implementing a national burden of disease study* (pp. 82–99). New York: Harvard Centre for Population and Development Studies.

Paúl, C., Fonseca, A. M., Martín, I., & Amado, J. (2005). Satisfação e qualidade de vida em idosos portugueses. *Psicologia, Saúde & Doenças, 7(1)*, 137–143.

Pereira, A., Izquierdo, M., Silva, A.J., Costa, A.M., Bastos, E., Gonzalez-Badillo J.J., & Marques, M.C. (2012). Effects of high-speed power training on functional capacity and muscle performance in older women. *Experimental Gerontology, 47*, 250–255.

Pibernik-Okanović, M. (2001). Psychometric properties of the World Health Organisation quality of life questionnaire (WHOQOL-100) in diabetic patients in Croatia. *Diabetes Research and Clinical Practice, 51*(2), 133–143. http://doi.org/10.1016/S0168-8227(00)00230-8.

Pimentel, F.L. (2006). *Qualidade de Vida e Oncologia.* Porto: Almedina.

Ploughman, M., McCarthy, J., Bosse, M., Sullivan, H.J., & Corbett, D. (2008). Does treadmill exercise improve performance of cognitive or upper-extremity tasks in people with chronic stroke? A randomized cross-over trial. *Archives of Physical Medicine and Rehabilitation, 89*, 2041–2047.

Revicki, A.D. (1993). Health care technology assessment and health-related quality of life. In D.H. Banta & B.R. Luci (Eds.). *Health care technology and its assessment: an international perspective* (pp. 115–131). New York: Oxford University Press;.

Rizzuto, D., Melis, R.J.F., Angleman, S., Qiu, C., & Marengoni, A. (2017). Effect of chronic diseases and multimorbidity on survival and functioning in elderly adults. *Journal of the American Geriatric Society, 65*(5), 1056–1060. doi: 10.1111/jgs.14868.

Rochon, P.A., & Gurwitz, J.H. (2017). The prescribing cascade revisited. *Lancet, 389*(10081), 1778–1780. doi: 10.1016/S0140-6736(17)31188-1.

Romero, M., Vivas-Consuelo, D., & Alvis-Guzman, N. (2013). Is Health Related Quality of Life (HRQoL) a valid indicator for health systems evaluation? *SpringerPlus, 2*(1), 664.

Rubenstein, L.Z., Harker, J.O., Salva, A., Guigoz, Y., & Vellas, B. (2001). Screening for undernutrition in geriatric practice: Developing the short-form Mini Nutritional Assessment (MNA-SF). *Journal of Gerontology, 56*, 366–377.

Ruivo, J.A. & Alcântara, P. (2012). Hipertensão arterial e exercício físico. *Revista Portuguesa de Cardiologia, 31*, 151–158.

Santos, C., Almeida, A., & Rosado, L. (2016). *Tradução, Adaptação Cultural e Validação do Questionário Quality of Life in Epilepsy (QOLIE-89) para a População Portuguesa,* Dissertação de Mestrado em Gestão de Unidades de Saúde, Universidade da Beira Interior, Faculdade de Ciências Sociais e Humanas, Covilhã.

Schwartzmann, L. (2007). Calidad de vida relacionada con la salud: aspectos conceptuales. *Cienc. enfermo dic., 9*(2), 9–21. www.scielo.d/sciel0.php?script=sci art text&pid=S071795532003000200002&lng=es&mm=iso.

Simões, A. (2005). "Envelhecer bem?—Um modelo." *Revista Portuguesa de Pedagogia, 1*, 217–227.

Small, B.J., Dixon, R.A., McArdle, J.J., & Grimm, K.J. (2012). Do changes in life-style engagement moderate cognitive decline in normal aging? Evidence from the Victoria Longitudinal Study. *Neuropsychology, 26,* 144–155. http://dx.doi.org/10.1037/a0026579.

Sousa, S., Pires, A., Conceição, C., Nascimento, T., Grenha, A., & Braz, L. (2011). Polimedicação em doentes idosos: adesão à terapêutica. *Revista Portuguesa Clínica Geral, 27,* 176–182.

Strehblow, C., Smeikal, M., & Fasching, P. (2014). Polypharmacy and excessive polypharmacy in octogenarians and older acutely hospitalized patients. *Wien Klin Wochenschr, 126*(7–8), 195–200. doi: 10.1007/s00508-013-0485-1.

Toscano, J.J.O. & Oliveira, A.C.C. (2009). Qualidade de Vidaem Idosos com distintos níveis de actividade física. *Revista Brasileira Med Esporte, 15*(3), 169–173.

Vancampfort, D., Mitchell, A.J., De Hert, M., Sienaert, P., Probst, M., Buys, R., & Stubbs, B. (2015). Prevalence and predictors of type 2 diabetes in people with bipolar disorder: a systematic review and meta-analysis. *Journal of Clinical Psychiatry, 76*(11), 1490–1499.

Van der Waal, J.M., Terwee, B.C., van der Windt, D.A., Bouter, L.M., & Dekker, J. (2005). The impact of non-traumatic hip and knee disorders on health-related quality of life as measured with the SF-36 or SF-12: a systematic review. *Quality of Life Research, 14,* 1141–1155.

Wagner, L.I., Beaumont, J.L., Ding, B., Malin, J., Peterman, A., Calhoun, F., & Cella, D. (2008). Measuring health-related quality of life and neutropenia-specific concerns among older adults undergoing chemotherapy: validation of the Functional Assessment of Cancer Therapy-Neutropenia (FACT-N). *Support Care Cancer, 16,* 47–56.

WHOQOL Group. (1995). The World Health Organization Quality of Life Assessment (WHOQOL): Position paper from the WHO. *Social Science and Medicine, 41*(10), 1403–1409.

World Health Organization (WHO) (1948). Construct of the World Health Organization basic document. Geneva, Switzerland: World Health Organization.

World Health Organization (WHO) (2002). "Active ageing. A policy framework." A contribution of WHO to the Second United Nations World Assembly on Aging. Madrid, Espanha, April.

World Health Organization (WHO) (2006). Constitution of The World Health Organization. *Basic Document Forthy-Fifth Edition,* 1–18. http://doi.org/12571729.

Wyles, H. & Rehman, H. (2005). Inappropriate polypharmacy in the elderly. *European Journal of Internal Medicine, 16*(5), 311–313.

Chapter 4

Functional characteristics of older adults in Mexico and Latin America

Health promotion programs

Oswaldo Ceballos-Gurrola,
Norma Angélica Borbón, Magdalena Soledad Chavero,
Nancy Cristina Banda Sauceda, Martha Ornelas,
Rosa Olivia Méndez, and Rosa María Cruz Castruita

Introduction

The purpose of this chapter is to provide information on the functional characteristics of older adults in Mexico and Latin America. It also provides ways they can be served through health promotion programs based on theoretical models that allow an integral evaluation of the functional capacity of the older adult through a set of variables that directly influences recovery, maintenance and functional improvement. Additionally, it provides information on the design and implementation of health promotion programs based on physical activity to enhance healthy physical condition.

The older adult (AM in Spanish) is defined as "a complex and multidimensional human whose well-being is influenced by different aspects, not only economic ones, but also their health, family and social support, level of functionality, degree of participation in society and their life history, among other factors" (Fernández-Ballesteros, 2009, 21). In Mexico, as in other Latin American countries such as Chile and Colombia, older persons are considered over 60 years old (Borba et al., 2008; Correa et al., 2011; García et al., 2013), unlike many developed countries, where the age of the older adult starts at age 65 (Huenchuan, 2013).

Population aging in Mexico and Latin America

One of the most worrying conditions in today's society is the accelerated aging of the population, where changes in population structures in both more developed and less developed countries have been largely encouraged by demographic transition, which is expected to continue changing in the years ahead (Lee & Donehower, 2010). The social transformation that this process has caused is related to decreasing population growth and greater life expectancy. Numbers are alarming in Mexico and Latin America. It is estimated that the number of older adults increases more significantly, unlike other regions of the world where in 2010 the proportion of older adults was 36 per 100 children. It is estimated that by 2036 this relationship will be reversed (Huenchuan, 2013), thereby causing the need for environmental adjustments to meet demands in terms of social security, equipment, infrastructure, and support programs (Sánchez, 2015).

The aging pace of Mexico and Latin America is even faster than it has been historically in developed countries. In the cases of Chile and Colombia, the aging stage began in 1960, causing changes in the structure of its population as well as in the causes of disease and death (Gajardo & Monsalves, 2013). In Columbia, however, a predominance in the population of 60+ over the population under 15 years old is expected by 2040 (Flórez et al., 2015). Unlike Paraguay, the overall fertility rate is still high (Red de Envejecimiento de la Asociación Latinoamericana de Población, 2011). Another country with high aging rates is Cuba, where people 60+ represent 16 per cent of the population and only 18.4 per cent are under 15 years of age (Domínguez-Alonso & Zaca, 2011). This is similar to Uruguay, where older adults represent 19 per cent of the total population (Paredes et al., 2010).

For Brazil, Peru, and Guatemala, the figures of the older population will be lower than those predicted for Mexico (Aguila et al., 2011), where an increase of 2 million by 2050 is estimated (World Health Organization (WHO), 2014), which is equivalent to 9.06 per cent of the total national population (García et al., 2013). Demographic changes in Mexico have responded to the profound social, political, and economic transformations that Mexican society has undergone in the last 100 years. All this is modulated by scientific and technological changes as part of the social and economic transformations along with the rest of the world (Pelcastre-Villafuerte et al., 2011).

Functionality in the older adult population

Aging is a process that involves changes in the biological, psychological, and social spheres, which impact on the quality of life due to limitations at the functional level (Ceballos, 2012). Therefore, evaluating the functional physical capacity of the older adult involves measuring the outcome of various biological, psychological, and social variables. Identifying functionality, not as one single element but in a holistic way, is necessary to recognize the levels of disability and dependence of the older adult. Functionality is also related to disease and its severity, as well as its influence on the physical state, cognition, mood, motivation to improve, and personal expectations (Segovia & Torres, 2011).

The most important changes in the *biological* sphere related to functional capacity are:

decreased muscle mass, strength, and function, known as sarcopenia (Paladines et al., 2016). This has a multifactorial origin and may include decreased physical activity, impaired endocrine function, chronic disease, resistance to insulin as well as nutritional deficiencies (Fielding, et al., 2011). Alterations to the locomotive apparatus produce impairment of the osseous system, giving rise to osteoporosis and eventually osteoarthritis. Diseases like the latter may become highly disabling due to decreased bone mineral density in this age group, increased brittleness and susceptibility to fractures.

(Tobías et al., 2014)

The modifications of aging in the biological sphere relate to the socio-medical sphere, where the work stage ends between the ages of 60 and 65, and the illness frequency increases in relation to previous stages of life. A progressive deterioration of physical and cognitive capacities occurs and there is loss of autonomy. These factors can cause anxiety, social isolation, and the appearance of depressive symptoms; if permanent, and the signs and symptoms increase, they can have an impact on health (Matutti & Tipismana, 2016) and consequently on the functionality of the older adult.

Among the changes in the *psychological* area, alterations of the neuro-motor system from aging of the nervous system are occurring, as evidenced by the loss of neurons, dendrites, enzymes, and receptors. Also, a reduction of catecholynergic and dopaminergic neurotransmitters takes place. This partially explains the cognitive decline (memory, concentration, attention, visuo-spatial ability, conceptualization, general intelligence) and failures in coordination of movements, which frequently occur. Likewise, postural reflexes decrease, thus resulting in instability and increased risk of falls (Penny & Melgar, 2012).

Aging is also a *social* process. The most notable change in family structure is the loss of spouse (widowhood), a more pronounced experience in women as they generally survive their husbands (Del Pozo & Thumala, 2016). For Castellanos and López (2010), seniority in Latin America is generally related to the withdrawal of social life. Older adults are vulnerable to dependency as a consequence of chronic diseases, motor or mental disabilities. This eventually increases the consumption of up to 50 per cent more health-related resources in families with at least one older adult, due to the presence of chronic pathologies (Manrique-Espinoza et al., 2013). In addition, a dependent older adult represents a responsibility mainly for their sons and daughters, with occasional participation of grandchildren and siblings (Bazo, 2008).

The loss of functionality in the older adult is linked to the decrease in the physiological function of many organs and systems, to the genetic information inherited from the parents, and to lifestyle throughout their life span. Furthermore, the social context is an important situation to consider, because it relates to adverse health events (falls, hospitalization, institutionalization, death) and with disability or dependency (Ávila-Funes et al., 2008).

Functional characteristics of older adults in Mexico and Latin America

In Mexico, one in four older adults is limited to basic and instrumental activities of daily living (Gutiérrez et al., 2012; Manrique-Espinoza et al., 2013) and about 84.9 per cent are dependent and have motor impairment (Pinillos-Patiño & Prieto-Suarez, 2012); they are associated with dependence, age, and marital status such as widow, divorcee, or single (Zavala-González & Domínguez-Sosa, 2011). These statistics relate to the high incidence of falls and fractures, which constitute one of the most important geriatric syndromes that cause loss of functionality. Also, advanced age is considered the second cause of disability (Instituto Nacional de Estadística y Geografía, 2010). According to figures from the Ministry of Health (Secretaría de Salud, 2011), prevalences increase in relation to age: at 60 years, 10.4 per cent to 18.7 per cent of men and women, respectively, suffer from a disability; while, in the 80- and 90-year-old groups, 38.7 per cent to 60 per cent of men and 48.3 per cent to 66 per cent of women suffer from these, respectively.

A study carried out with the Colombian population indicates that 52.6 per cent of older adults present mild cognitive impairment, 39.6 per cent moderate impairment, and 7.8 per cent severe impairment. On the other hand, 73.9 per cent of older adults are independent in the development of basic activities of daily living, and only 26.1 per cent are dependent on some activities. The loss of functionality is associated with age, the presence of chronic diseases, and multiple usage of drugs. Likewise, living with a partner and children contributes to the maintenance of functionality by being considered a protective factor; this is not the case with the presence of depressive states, which have a direct impact on the physical health of the elderly and contribute to social isolation (Villarreal & Month, 2012).

Results of a study conducted in Brazil indicate that the functionality of older adults is affected by high frequency of falls; its main causes are attributed to impaired balance, muscle weakness, and the feeling of dizziness. As a result, 15 per cent of older adults who suffered a fall become affected in their functionality, because the independent performance of some basic activities of daily life is compromised. With regard to psychological and socio-cultural factors, results indicate the presence of depressive states in 6.3 per cent of the cases after having suffered a fall. Likewise, a correlation was found between the decrease in functional independence and age, in which no correlation was found on functional independence (Fhon et al., 2012).

In the case of Cuba, the dependence and independence of the older adult is not associated with gender. However, the prevalence of chronic diseases—although affecting the total population—is more pronounced among females, where main diseases are arterial hypertension, diabetes mellitus, and ischemic heart disease (García et al., 2010). Concerning the difficulties shown by older adults to perform instrumental activities of daily living, it was found that the greatest number of associated variables is present in seven cities in Latin America: Brazil, Cuba, Uruguay, Chile, Argentina, Mexico, and Barbados. In all cities there is an association between the difficulty to carry out instrumental activities of daily life and age, gender, chronic diseases, depressive states, cataloging one's health status as bad, and cognitive impairment. It is important to note that in Chile and Argentina, a higher level of education was associated with a lower frequency of disability (Menéndez et al., 2014).

In sum, the functionality of the older adult in various countries of Mexico and Latin America is compromised, not only by the age factor and the natural biological changes that occur during the aging process, but by several factors that influence the maintenance of autonomy. Although physiological changes have a great influence, so has the suffering of chronic diseases, the presence of depression, as well as multiple socio-cultural factors. Thus, the evaluation of the older adult requires an integral approach taking the functional physical evaluation into account, and also those variables that affect functionality, and therefore one's independence and health.

Theoretical models in the design of health promotion programs

Researchers indicate that health and public health promotion programs that are based on models or theories of the social and behavioral sciences are more effective than those lacking theoretical basis. Programs should not only be directed at people, but should also consider interpersonal, organizational, and environmental factors that influence health behavior (de Silva et al., 2014; Glanz & Bishop, 2010; Glanz et al., 2008). Thus, it can be inferred that the use of models or theories helps to describe aspects that deal with the determinants necessary to achieve a change in lifestyle (Bartholomew et al., 2011).

A theory is mandatory to guide, plan, implement, and evaluate health promotion programs. It indicates which variables are important for intervention and which variables need change to achieve effective intervention (Lippke & Ziegelmann, 2008). Furthermore, these variables avoid errors when no effectiveness is found in the program due to inadequate design or implementation (Bartholomew et al., 2011); they help to predict and explain phenomena and can be used to formulate testable hypotheses

(Prochaska et al., 2008). Studies conducted in Mexico are based on the *Health Promotion Model* (Pender, Murdaugh, & Parsons, 2011) and the *Toronto Physical Condition, Physical Activity and Health Model* for health promoting physical activity in older adults.

The *Health Promotion Model* allows the understanding of human behaviors related to health and, in turn, works as a guide for the generation of healthy behaviors (Pender, Murdaugh, & Parsons, 2011, 44 and 61). This model seeks to illustrate the multi-faceted nature of people in their interaction with the environment when they strive for a desired state of health. It characterizes biological, psychological, and socio-cultural factors, which are predictive of certain behavior; and it emphasizes the link between personal characteristics, experiences, knowledge, beliefs, and situational aspects associated with the behaviors or health behaviors that are intended to be achieved (Aristizábal et al., 2011). This model has been used in the field of physical activity for different types of population (see Burke et al., 2012; Fitzpatrick et al., 2008), where the promotion of health through programs directed to the elderly has positively influenced their levels of physical activity, and thus, has a beneficial impact on people and their health.

The *Health Promotion Model* consists of nine concepts that fall into the following three categories: (1) individual characteristics and experiences including personal, biological, psychological and socio-cultural factors; (2) specific cognitions of behavior and affection; and (3) behavioral result represented by health promotion behavior. The first category is related to the variables that influence the functionality of the older adult (Aristizábal et al., 2011).

On the other hand, the *Toronto Physical Activity and Health Model* focuses on a healthy physical condition, which influences the health status of people and reciprocally their engagement in physical activity. A healthy physical condition is related to genetic inheritance and other factors, such as lifestyle, personal, social, and environmental aspects that will determine the optimization of a healthy physical condition (Blázquez, 2015).

The *Toronto Model* is composed of five variables:

- physical activity that includes the components of leisure physical activity, physical activity of occupation and physical activity related to the tasks;
- healthy physical condition that includes the morphological, muscular, motor, cardiorespiratory and metabolic components;
- health that deals with aspects related to quality of life, morbidity, and mortality;
- genetics; and
- other factors that include lifestyle, personal aspects, social aspects, and environment.

All these components will act together to enhance the health improvements provided by the healthy physical condition and, in turn, the functionality and general health of the older adult.

Promotion of health through programs of physical activity

In older adults, functional limitations progress naturally over time, especially for older adults with lower levels of physical activity (Phillips, 2015). This is because from the age of 65, the loss of functional capacity is estimated to occur about 10 per cent after each decade. A decrease in bone mineral density already starts to take place from the age of 35 (Tobías et al., 2014), which is even more pronounced in adults older than 70 (Riera-Espinoza, 2009).

For many years, physical activity has been considered as one of the fundamental pillars in the integral overall development of people, emphasizing its playful, integrative character and its direct influence on the maintenance of health (Michelini, 2013). The objectives of healthy physical activity is: to improve the healthy physical condition; to reduce the effects of aging at the motor, physiological and mental level; to maintain basic safety and health measures in their execution; and to create habits associated with physical exercise and an active and healthy lifestyle (Casimiro et al., 2014).

For senior citizens, the practice of physical activity also has great social importance because it facilitates the prevention, treatment, and rehabilitation of various diseases (Ceballos, 2012); it contributes to the maintenance of a good quality of life (Heyward, 2008); and it relates to increased longevity (Organización Mundial de la Salud (OMS), 2015a). However, health-related improvements will depend on the dose-response relationship, which is characterized by volume, intensity, frequency, type of exercise, and rest. All of these will determine the impact of the benefits, reducing in turn risk factors that compromise health due to inadequate dose and control (Yen-Chun et al., 2011).

Physical activity recommendations for adults 65 and older issued by the OMS (2015b) indicate that older adults should perform at least 150 minutes of moderate-intensity physical activity with a frequency of at least 5 days per week, or perform at least 75 minutes of aerobic physical activity at vigorous intensity, or a combination of both. Types of physical activity can include leisure activities, transportation, work, household tasks, sports, or exercise. The emphasis of physical activity shall be aerobic and be performed for intermittent periods of 10 minutes in length in order to achieve the recommended minimum distributed throughout the week. To achieve better benefits, older adults shall increase the volume to 300 minutes per week at moderate intensity or 150 minutes per week at vigorous intensity.

Physical activity programs involving older adults with low mobility should include coordination, agility, and strength, to improve balance and prevent falls; frequency must be at least 3 days a week. Also, muscle strengthening programs should be performed at least 2 days per week and include the use of large muscle groups (OMS, 2015c). Older adults with serious physical limitations who cannot meet the minimum recommendation should perform as much physical activity as possible based on their health conditions (González-Gross & Meléndez, 2013). A systemic physical activity will promote significant benefits and reduce functional and mobility limitations as well as the risk of disability (von Bonsdorff et al., 2008).

The American College of Sports Medicine (ACSM, 2013) indicates that the physical activity prescription for most adults should be of moderate intensity and with rhythmic aerobic exercises—using large muscle groups and with aerobic predominance. The prescription of physical exercise must indicate the type of activity, mode, intensity, volume, frequency, and rest. All these are important variables to adequately structure the exercise sessions and to fulfill the objectives to be achieved with their practice (Márquez & Garatachea, 2013).

Healthy physical condition in the older adult

Physical condition is defined as the set of organic, anatomical, and physiological qualities or conditions that a person must meet to be able to carry out physical efforts, whether it is in daily life or in sports (Fernández, 2009). Today, physical condition represents the body's potential to face physical challenges and can be defined as the weighted sum of the different physical capacities of a person (Ros, 2011).

The *Toronto Physical Condition, Physical Activity, and Health Model* points to very specific goals: the improvements in healthy physical fitness and health status that allow people to autonomously carry out daily activities and perform physical tasks without excessive fatigue, enjoy active leisure time, avoid motor ailments, and enhance the intellectual ability (Escalante, 2011). Two main physiological adaptations are established that will be based on the levels of physical activity. The first one emphasizes health through improvements in the components of cardiorespiratory endurance, muscular endurance, muscle strength, body composition, and flexibility. The second is linked to sports performance where improvements in agility, balance, coordination, speed, power, and reaction time are accentuated.

Proper physical conditions for individuals are obtained as part of healthy lifestyles, depending upon the health status, age, and initial physical condition. According to Pancorbo (2008), the components of fitness are associated with physiological improvements that allow good health and disease prevention—and not necessarily with athletic performance. Therefore, even if a person does not have the physical constitution that allows for optimum sport performance, one can still enjoy a good health-related physical condition by engaging in regular physical activity, which affects body composition and the overall aerobic capacity (Ros, 2011). For the senior population, the importance of optimizing healthy physical condition lies in the preventive approach to diseases, which implies improving the functionality and health status of the individual.

According to Ros (2011), there are three fundamental physical capacities in the field of health: aerobic endurance, strength, and flexibility. Aerobic resistance is paramount in any program of physical activity because of the adaptations at the metabolic, cardiovascular, and cardiorespiratory level it produces. Strength and flexibility are essential for proper functioning of the musculoskeletal system, as well as coordination and balance, which directly influence the maintenance of posture, correct ambulation, and the execution of complex movements. Therefore, the development of these capacities is key in the prevention and improvement of health, which directly affect the quality of life. The healthy physical condition includes the following advantages: (1) improvement of the efficiency and reduction of fatigue when performing daily activities; (2) disease prevention related to lack of movement; (3) promotion of enjoyment of leisure time; (4) improvement of self-esteem and promotion of interpersonal relationships; and (5) improvement in brain function. Physical activity programs can be effective in maintaining the health of the older adults, as well as in preventing obesity, diabetes, and hypertension.

Conclusion

This chapter reinforces the knowledge that when older adults participate regularly in physical exercise programs, positive adaptations occur that improve body composition, cardiovascular functioning, and motor abilities. When combining these physical activity programs with adequate diets, the effects are even better, in that they influence the psychological state and the improvement of biological markers.

In Mexico, unfortunately, many physical activity programs available to citizens are rarely planned or structured, and they often lack a clear scientific support. The differences and benefits between the *structured and nonstructured* programs, then, are immense. The structured programs that are supported and evaluated based on theoretical models emphasize the adaptation of facilitating environments to enhance people's adhesion to an active lifestyle. And structured models also explain the causal relationship between the program and the desired results.

References

Aguila, E., Díaz, C., Fu, M. M., Kapteyn, A., & Pierson, A. (2011). *Envejecer en México: Condiciones de Vida y Salud*. México: AARP, RAND Corporation, Centro FOX. ISBN: 978-8330-5945-1.

American College of Sports Medicine (ACSM). (2013). *ACSM's guidelines for exercise testing and prescription*. Baltimore, MD: Lippincott Williams & Wilkins.

Aristizábal, G. P., Blanco, D. M., Sánchez, A., & Ostiguín, R. M. (2011). El modelo de promoción de la salud de Nola Pender. Una reflexión en torno a su comprensión. *Enfermería Universitaria, 8*(4), 16–23.

Ávila-Funes, J. A., Aguilar-Navarro, S., & Melano-Carranza, E. (2008). La fragilidad, concepto enigmático y controvertido de la geriatría: la visión biológica. *Gaceta Médica de México, 144*(3), 255–262.

Bartholomew, L. K., Parcel, G. S., Kok, G., & Gottlieb, N. H. (2011). *Planning health promotion programmes: an intervention mapping approach*. Hoboken, NJ: John Wiley & Sons.

Bazo, M. T. (2008). Personas mayores y solidaridad familiar. *Política y sociedad, 45*(2), 73–85.

Blázquez, M. J. (2015). *La actividad física con caballos como medio terapéutico para mejorar la capacidad funcional y la calidad de vida de las personas de la tercera edad y de las afectadas por el síndrome de fibromialgia: el método centauro como programmea formativo de intervención* (Thesis doctoral). Retrieved from www.tdx.cesca.cat/handle/10803/297703?show=full.

Borba, R., Santa, M. A. C., Borges, P. R., Corrêa, J., & González, C. (2008). Medidas de estimación de la estatura aplicadas al índice de masa corporal (IMC) en la evaluación del estado nutricional de adultos mayores. *Revista Chilena de Nutrición, 35*(1), 272–279. doi: 10.4067/S0717-75182008000400003.

Burke, L., Lee, A. H., Pasalich, M., Jancey, J., Kerr, D., & Howat, P. (2012). Effects of a physical activity and nutrition programme for seniors on body mass index and waist-to-hip ratio: a randomised controlled trial. *Preventive medicine, 54*(6), 397–401.

Casimiro, A. J., Delgado, M., & Águila, C. (2014). *Actividad física, educación y salud*. Editorial Universidad de Almería.

Castellanos, F. & López, A. L. (2010). Mirando pasar la vida desde la ventana: significado de la vejez y la discapacidad de un grupo de ancianos en un contexto de pobreza. *Investigación en Enfermería: Imagen y Desarrollo, 12*(2), 37–53.

Ceballos, O. (2012). *Actividad física en el adulto mayor*. México: Manual moderno.

Correa, B. J. E., Gámez, M. E. R., Ibáñez, P. M., & Rodríguez, D. K. D. (2011). Aptitud física en mujeres adultas mayores vinculadas a un programmea de envejecimiento activo. *Salud UIS, 43*(3), 263–269.

Del Pozo, M. T. & Thumala, D. (2016). Reconstrucción de soportes sociales en mujeres urbanos populares post viudez: Una mirada a los cuidados. *Psicoperspectivas, 15*(3), 78–86. doi:10.5027/psicoperspectivas-Vol.15-Issue3-fulltext-753.

De Silva, M. J., Breuer, E., Lee, L., Asher, L., Chowdhary, N., Lund, C., & Patel, V. (2014). Theory of change: a theory-driven approach to enhance the Medical Research Council's framework for complex interventions. *Trials, 15*(1), 267–279. doi:10.1186/1745-6215-15-267.

Domínguez-Alonso, E. & Zacca, E. (2011). Sistema de salud de Cuba. *Salud pública de México*, *53*, s168–s176.

Escalante, Y. (2011). Physical activity, exercise, and fitness in the public health field. *Rev Esp Salud Pública*, *84*(4), 325–328.

Fernández, J. M. (2009). *Valoración de la condición física del alumno del CEIP o grupo de Ribeira mediante la batería Eurofit*. London: Lulu Enterprises.

Fernández-Ballesteros, R. (2009). *Envejecimiento Activo: Contribuciones a la Psicología* (p. 21). Madrid: Editorial Pirámide.

Fhon, J. R. S., Fabrício-Wehbe, S. C. C., Vendruscolo, T. R. P., Stackfleth, R., Marques, S., & Rodrigues, R. A. P. (2012). Accidental falls in the elderly and their relation to functional capacity. *Revista latino-americana de enfermagem*, *20*(5), 927–934.

Fielding, R. A., Vellas, B., Evans, W. J., Bhasin, S., Morley, J. E., Newman, A. B., ... & Zamboni, M. (2011). Sarcopenia: an undiagnosed condition in older adults. Current consensus definition: prevalence, etiology, and consequences. International working group on sarcopenia. *Journal of the American Medical Directors Association*, *12*(4), 249–256.

Fitzpatrick, S. F., Reddy, S., Lommel, T. S., Fischer, J. G., Speer, E. M., Stephens, H., Park, S., & Johnson, M. A. (2008). Physical activity and physical function improved following a community-based intervention in older adults in Georgia senior centers. *Journal of Nutrition for the Elderly*, *27*(1–2), 135–154.

Flórez, C. E., Villar, L., Puerta, N., & Berrocal, L. (2015). *El proceso de envejecimiento de la población en Colombia: 1985–2050: Fundación Saldarriaga Concha*. Bogotá, D.C. Colombia, 67.

Gajardo, J. & Monsalves, M. J. (2013). Demencia, un tema urgente para Chile. *Revista Chilena de Salud Pública*,*17*(1), 22–25.

García, M., García, M., García, R., & Taño, L. (2010). Salud funcional y enfermedades generales asociadas en ancianos. *Revista de Ciencias Médicas de Pinar del Río*,*14*(1), 128–137.

García, S. G., Pérez, M. D. L. L. V., Rodríguez, A. R. T., & Pantoja, J. E. G. (2013). Fortalecimiento de la atención primaria del adulto mayor ante la transición demográfica en México. *Atención Primaria*, *45*(5), 231–232.

Glanz, K. & Bishop, D. B. (2010). The role of behavioural science theory in development and implementation of public health interventions. *Annual Review of Public Health*, *31*(1), 399–418.

Glanz, K., Rimer, B. K., & Viswanath, K. (2008). Health behaviour and health education. *Theory, Research and Practice* (4th ed.). San Francisco, CA: Jossey Bass.

González-Gross, M. & Meléndez, A. (2013). Sedentarism, active lifestyle and sport: impact on health and obesity prevention. *Nutrición Hospitalaria*, *28*(5), 89–98. doi:10.3305/nh.2013.28.sup5.6869.

Gutiérrez, J. P., Rivera-Dommarco, J., Shamah-Levy, T., Villalpando-Hernández, S., Franco, S., Cuevas-Nasu, L., & Hernández-Ávila, M. (2012). Encuesta Nacional de Salud y Nutrición 2012. *Resultados Nacionales. Cuernavaca, México: Instituto Nacional de Salud Pública* (MX), 2012. Retrieved from http://ensanut.insp.mx/informes/ENSANUT2012ResultadosNacionales.pdf.

Heyward, V. H. (2008). *Evaluación de la aptitud física y prescripción del ejercicio*. Madrid, España: Editorial Médica Panamericana S.A.

Huenchuan, S. (2013). *Envejecimiento, solidaridad y protección social en América Latina y el Caribe: La hora de avanzar hacia la igualdad.* Santiago de Chile: CEPAL.

Instituto Nacional de Estadística y Geografía. (2010). Hombres y mujeres en México 2010. Retrieved from www.inegi.org.mx/prod_serv/contenidos/espanol/bvinegi/productos/integracion/sociodemografico/mujeresyhombres/2010/MyH_2010.pdf.

Lee, R. & Donehower, G. S. (2010). El envejecimiento de la poblaciòn, las transferencias intergenaracionales y el crecimiento económico: Amércia Latina en el contexto mundial. *Notas de Poblaión, 90,* 13–37.

Lippke, S. & Ziegelmann, J. P. (2008). Theory-based health behaviour change: developing, testing, and applying theories for evidence-based interventions. *Applied Psychology, 57*(4), 698–716. doi:10.1111/j.1464-0597.2008.00339.x.

Manrique-Espinoza, B., Salinas-Rodríguez, A., Moreno-Tamayo, K. M., Acosta-Castillo, I., Sosa-Ortiz, A. L., Gutiérrez-Robledo, L. M., & Téllez-Rojo, M. M. (2013). Health conditions and functional status of older adults in Mexico. *Salud pública de México, 55*(Suppl. 2), S323–S331.

Márquez, R. & Garatachea, N. (2013). *Actividad física y salud.* Madrid: Ediciones Díaz de Santos.

Matutti, M. & Tipismana, O. (2016). Prevalencia de depresión mayor en adultos mayores atendidos ambulatoriamente en un hospital de lima metropolitana. *Interacciones, 2*(2), 171–187.

Menéndez, J., Guevara, A., Arcia, N., León, E. M., Marín, C., & Alfonso, J. C. (2014). Enfermedades crónicas y limitación funcional en adultos mayores. Estudio comparativo en siete ciudades de América Latina y el Caribe. *Revista Panamericana de Salud Publica, 17*(5/6), 353–361.

Michelini, E. (2013). *The role of sport in health-related promotion of physical activity: the perspective of the health system.* Springer. doi:10.1007/978-3-658-08188-1.

Organización Mundial de la Salud (OMS). (2015a). Enfermedades no transmisibles. Retrieved from www.who.int/mediacentre/factsheets/fs355/es/.

Organización Mundial de la Salud (OMS). (2015b). Informe mundial sobre envejecimiento y salud. Retrieved from www.who.int/ageing/publications/world-report-2015/es/.

Organización Mundial de la Salud (OMS). (2015c). Physical activity and older adults. Recommended levels of physical activity for adults aged 65 and above. Retrieved from www.who.int/dietphysicalactivity/factsheet_olderadults/en/.

Paladines, B., Quizhpi, M., & Villota, P. (2016). Tratamiento integral de la sarcopenia senil. *Revista de la Facultad de Ciencias Químicas, Edición Especial, (ed. especial),* 41–48. Ecuador: Universidad de Cuenca.

Pancorbo, S. A. E. (2008). *Medicina y ciencias del deporte y la actividad física* (vol. 1). México, DF.: OCEANO/ergon.

Paredes, M., Ciarniello, M., & Brunet, N. (2010). *Indicadores sociodemográficos de envejecimiento y vejez en Uruguay.* Uruguay: Lucida ediciones. ISBN: 978-9974-0-0668-3.

Pelcastre-Villafuerte, B. E., Treviño-Siller, S., González-Vázquez, T., & Márquez-Serrano, M. (2011). Apoyo social y condiciones de vida de adultos mayores que viven en la pobreza urbana en México. *Cadernos de Saúde Pública*, 27(3), 460–470.

Pender, N. J., Murdaugh, C. L., & Parsons, M. A. (2011). *Health promotion in nursing practice* (6th ed.). Upper Saddler River, NJ: Prentice Hall.

Penny, E. & Melgar, F. (2012). Cambios anatómicos y fisiológicos durante el envejecimiento y su impacto clínico. In E. Peny (Ed.), *Geriatría y Gerontología para el médico internista* (pp. 37–56). Bolivia: La Hoguera.

Phillips, L. J. (2015). Retirement community residents' physical activity, depressive symptoms, and functional limitations. *Clinical Nursing Research*, 24(1), 7–28. doi:10.1177/1054773813508133.

Pinillos-Patiño, Y. & Prieto-Suárez, E. (2012). Funcionalidad física de personas mayores institucionalizadas y no institucionalizadas en Barranquilla, Colombia. *Revista de Salud Pública*, 14(3), 436–445.

Prochaska, J. O., Wright, J. A., & Velicer, W. F. (2008). Evaluating theories of health behaviour change: a hierarchy of criteria applied to the transtheoretical model. *Applied Psychology*, 57(4), 561–588. doi:10.1111/j.1464-0597.2008.00345.x.

Red de Envejecimiento de la Asociación Latinoamericana de Población (2011) Envejecimiento poblacional y condiciones de vida de los adultos mayores. La situación paraguaya en perspectiva latinoamericana. *Perspectivas Sociales*, 14(2), 47–68.

Riera-Espinoza, G. (2009). Epidemiología de la osteoporosis en Latino América. *Salud Pública de México*, 51(Suppl. 1), s52–s55.

Ros, J. A. (2011). *Actividad Física Ros Salud Hacia un Estilo de Vida Activo*. Murcia: Novograf. ISBN 978-84-96994-04-1. Retrieved from www.murciasalud. es/recursos/publicaciones/actividad_fisica_mas_salud.pdf.

Sánchez, G. (2015). Ambiente físico-social y envejecimiento de la población desde la gerontología ambiental y geografía: Implicaciones socioespaciales en América Latina. *Revista de Geografía Norte Grande*, (60), 97–114.

Secretaría de Salud. (2011). Perfil epidemiológico del adulto mayor en México 2010. Retrieved from www.epidemiologia.salud.gob.mx/doctos/infoepid/publicaciones/2011/monografias/P_EPI_DEL_ADULTO_MAYOR_EN_MEXICO_2010.pdf.

Segovia, M. G. & Torres, E. A. (2011). Funcionalidad del adulto mayor y el cuidado enfermero. *Gerokomos*, 22(4), 162–166.

Tobías, J. H., Gould, V., Brunton, L., Deere, K., Rittweger, J., Lipperts, M., & Grimm, B. (2014). Physical activity and bone: may the force be with you. *Frontiers In Endocrinology*, 5, 1–5. doi:10.3389/fendo.2014.00020.

Villarreal, G. & Month, E. (2012). Ondición sociofamiliar, asistencial y de funcionalidad del adulto mayor de 65 años en dos comunas de Sincelejo (Colombia). Salud Uninorte. *Barranquilla*, 28(1), 75–87.

Von Bonsdorff, M. B., Leinonen, R., Kujala, U. M., Heikkinen, E., Törmäkangas, T., Hirvensalo, M., & ... Rantanen, T. (2008). Effect of physical activity counseling on disability in older people: a 2-year randomized controlled trial. *Journal of the American Geriatrics Society*, 56(12), 2188–2194. doi:10.1111/j.1532-5415.2008.02000.x.

World Health Organization. (2014). *Estadísticas sanitarias mundiales 2014*. Recuperado de Retrieved from: http://apps.who.int/iris/bitstream/10665/131953/1/9789240692695_spa.pdf?ua=1.

Yen-Chun, L., Lian-Hua, H., Mei, Ch. Y., & John, J. T. (2011). Leisure-time physical activities for community older people with chronic diseases. *Journal of Clinical Nursing, 20*(7/8), 940–949. doi:10.1111/j.1365-2702.2009.02877.x.

Zavala-González, M. A. & Domínguez-Sosa, G. (2011). Funcionalidad para la vida diaria en adultos mayores. *Revista Médica del Instituto Mexicano del Seguro Social, 49*(6), 585–596.

Chapter 5

Aging in Ghana

A public health and cultural perspective

Delali Margaret Badasu, Richmond Aryeetey,
Bella Bello Bitugu, and Reginald Ocansey

Introduction

This chapter discusses the current situation of aging in Ghana, focusing on socio-demographic characteristics and the health situation with a cultural perspective. In Ghana, there are unwritten but traditionally established norms by which aging and its associated characteristics are integrated into societal living. These cultural norms, including respect for the aged and reciprocity of care between parent and offspring (in both the biological and social sense) have served the purpose of providing a social safety net within which the needs of the aged are provided.

Because of the modernizing processes of urbanization, migration, and exposure to external influences, these norms are being transformed, and rapidly so, in such a way that the traditional safety nets have been undermined. In the absence of appropriate interventions, the aged are likely to be more severely affected by lifestyle-determined non-communicable diseases and disabilities. The aged in Ghana need physical and emotional care as well as protection from abuse and an enabling environment that fosters a healthy and active lifestyle. Currently, public-funded services and civil society initiatives are far in between to meet these needs.

In addition to traditional home care, non-family-based informal as well as formal commercial care options for the aged are emerging. Private commercial or non-family care options are expected to complement the dwindling traditional family-based care norms. The aged in Ghana, therefore, have unmet need for care, and particularly in urban settings. Although a National Aging Policy exists, it is yet to translate into easily accessible funded programs that deliver support services for the aged in Ghana. This chapter discusses not only the current situation of the aged but also projects scenarios and options for aged care in the future that is based upon available evidence and best practices that are suited to the local norms and culture.

About the context of Ghana

The Republic of Ghana is a relatively small sized country (92,000 square miles) that is situated in West Africa, South of the Sahara. The World Bank classifies Ghana as a low middle-income country; the estimated Gross Domestic Product is US$37.5 billion. Ghana is counted among the few Sub-Saharan African countries which achieved significant progress in reducing income poverty by the Millennium Development Goals (MDGs) timeline of 2015; currently, 24.2 percent of the population are considered poor (The World Bank, 2017) and average per capita income status of the population is relatively low. According to the *2016 World Population Data Sheet*, published by the Population Reference Bureau (2016) with data from the World Bank, Ghana's Gross National Income (GNI) per capita in purchasing power parity (PPP) in 2015 was US$4,070.00 compared with an average of US$10,215.00 for developing countries (Population Reference Bureau, 2016).

Agriculture employs 45 percent of the economically active population of Ghana (Ghana Statistical Service (GSS), Ghana Health Service (GHS), & ICF International, 2015). In 2016, the United Nations Population Fund (UNFPA) estimated Ghana's population at 28 million people (UNFPA, 2016) with an annual average population growth rate of 2.4 percent. Typical of other countries in the Sub-Sahara Africa region, Ghana's population is young with close to two-fifths (39 percent) under 15 years and growing rapidly. But the growth of the population aged 60 years and over has also been rapid in recent decades, as in other developing countries. Population aging has been a global phenomenon and has been referred to as a demographic shift by the UNFPA. In Ghana, the population has also experienced rapid urbanization and more than half (54 percent) of the total national population now resides in urban areas (GSS, 2013).

In Ghana, the aged (adults 60 years and above) constitute 7.6 percent (see Figure 5.1) of household population (Ghana Statistical Service (GSS), Ghana Health Service (GHS), & ICF International, 2015). The trends (see Figure 5.2) over the last four decades, however, show that Ghana's aged population is growing at a rapid rate (GSS, 2013; Mba, 2010; Tawiah, 2011; World Health Organization (WHO), 2014). Recent demographic evidence indicates that the majority of the aged in Ghana are within the 60–74 years age bracket (Figure 5.1). Considering that fertility rate is declining (Total Fertility Rate (TFR)=6.4 in 1988, and 4.2 in 2014) (GSS, GHS, & ICF International, 2015) and life expectancy rate has been increasing (60 years for males and 63 years for females in 2016) (Population Reference Bureau, 2016), it can be expected that Ghana's population will continue to age rapidly. This means that the nation has to be prepared to support the aged with their unique health and social needs.

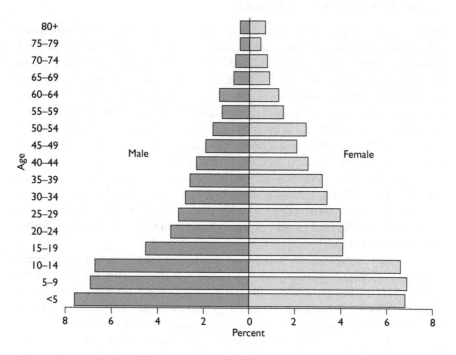

Figure 5.1 Overview of socio-demographic characteristics of the aged in Ghana.

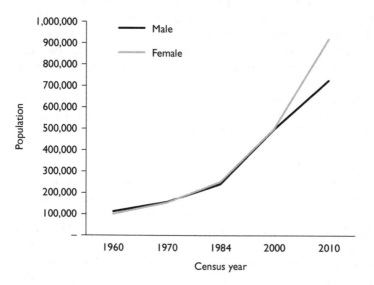

Figure 5.2 The growth of the male and female elderly population, 1960–2010.

An estimated 60 percent of the aged (60 years and over) live in rural areas (WHO, 2014). Some of those who migrate to live and/or work in urban areas tend to return to their rural home communities when they retire from employment as a coping mechanism against high costs of living in urban areas (Mba, 2010). Women are less likely than men to have formal education or to be in the high categories of wealth quintiles.

Less than 10 percent of Ghana's working population are wage earners. Therefore, the majority of the population do not benefit from a formal pension system upon retirement from work (GSS, 2013). Even among those who are eligible, pension benefits are generally minimal and highly depreciated by high rates of inflation. Eventually the benefits are insufficient in supporting the needs of most aged persons. It has been reported that, in Ghana, most people enter retirement with poverty and deprivation (Aboh & Ncama, 2017).

As a reflection of occupation in the general public, the majority of the aged in Ghana either are presently or have been working in agriculture/forestry industry as food crop farmers (63.1 percent) or harvesting food from forests. These rural dwelling farmers are likely to keep working the land in their old age until they can work no more. Some of them, therefore, depend heavily on other sources of livelihood, such as support from offspring, family, and remittances to meet their needs (Aikins & Apt, 2016).

Health and aging in Ghana

A rapid epidemiologic transition is occurring in Ghana and is having widespread adverse effects on the health of the aged. Although living longer, the aged are now living and coping with a high burden of non-communicable diseases (NCDs). Evidence from the 2005 WHO Global Aging and Adult Health survey (SAGE) indicates that the most common NCD challenges among the aged in Ghana include oral health problems (45 percent), hypertension (33 percent), arthritis (14 percent), and diabetes (7 percent) (Ayernor, 2012; WHO, 2014).

The challenge of NCDs in Ghana is by no means unique to the aged; it affects the younger population as well. However, among the aged, NCDs have a greater adverse impact due to their emotional, financial, and physical needs. Emergence of NCDs in Ghana has been linked with community-wide changes in diets and lifestyles (Dake, Tawiah, & Badasu, 2011; de-Graft Aikins, 2007).

About 40 percent of older persons reported various degrees of deficiencies in their capacity to perform daily activities (Ayernor, 2012). It has been reported that the aged in urban centers are more likely to die from falls and fall-related injuries. On the other hand, those in rural areas are living with a greater burden of injuries. These injuries are due mainly to agriculture and transportation. However, there are also concerns related to abandonment and abuse of the aged (WHO, 2014).

Another important health challenge of the aged in Ghana is disability. The 2010 population and household census reported that Ghanaians 60 years and older were six times more likely to report disability than those under 60 years (GSS, 2013). The major disabling conditions were related to impairments of the eye and limbs (Table 5.1). The high rates of disability among the aged affects their capacity for engaging in various activities including employment and income generation.

Disability also affects the quality of life of the aged and makes them dependent on others for care, especially when they do not have access to basic household amenities to support them to live a healthy and active life. For example, only 13 percent of aged in Ghana live in homes with toilet facility inside the residence (GSS, 2013); this situation increases their risk of falls that are linked with reduced functioning and wellbeing. An estimated 44 percent of aged respondents in the WHO SAGE study reported fall-related injury during the year preceding the study (Stewart Williams et al., 2015).

The aged in Ghana seek health care from either one or a combination of three health systems that co-exist in Ghana: conventional, traditional, and faith-based (Aryeetey, Aikins, Dako-Gyeke, & Adongo, 2015; de-Graft Aikins, 2007; de-Graft Aikins et al., 2010). Through the conventional health system, the aged who are 70 years and above receive free care for covered conditions under the National Health Insurance Scheme (NHIS) (Ministry of Health (MOH), 2004). A study conducted in 2011 and 2012 reported that this exemption policy is beneficial as the aged were more likely to be enrolled in the NHIS (Duku, van Dullemen, & Fenenga, 2015). The NHIS, however, does not cover the treatment of some of the NCDs that commonly afflict the aged. Also, specialized health care by gerontologists has been limited to the teaching hospitals and health care facilities that offer tertiary health services. Most of these specialist health facilities are found in urban areas. Meanwhile, the majority of the aged reside in rural areas and have limited or no physical access to the specialist health facilities.

Private care facilities have been important components of the health care system in Ghana, providing services that are priced quite a bit higher than public facilities. Some private facilities that provide services for the elderly are not eligible for reimbursement under the NHIS. Financial access to health services, thus, remains a major concern for the aged, particularly those with NCDs. Hence, a health care policy that includes aged persons in the 60–69 years category is necessary.

Table 5.1 Type and age distribution of disability among Ghanaians

Type of disability	0–59	60–64	65–69	70–74	75–79	80+	All
Sight	24.7	38.6	40.0	41.9	42.5	39.9	29.0
Hearing	10.5	9.6	9.8	11.1	11.5	14.1	10.8
Speech	11.8	5.9	5.2	4.4	4.0	4.3	9.9
Physical	15.9	23.1	24.4	25.2	26.1	26.4	18.4
Intellectual	12.9	6.8	6.2	5.3	4.8	5.7	11.0
Emotional	15.8	9.2	8.2	6.7	6.3	5.8	13.4
Other	8.4	6.7	6.3	5.5	4.8	3.9	7.5
Total	100.0	100.0	100.0	100.0	100.0	100.0	100.0
Number	745,552	51,137	37,324	59,728	41,936	84,958	1,020,635

Source: Ghana Statistical Service, 2013.

Aging in a Ghanaian cultural context

The aged in Ghana are exposed to a cultural environment within which they live and cope with multiple social, cultural, and traditional dynamics. These dynamics have implications for their health and wellbeing. A key dynamic in the situation of the aged in Ghana is their identity and how they are perceived. Ghanaian tradition typically venerates old age and ascribes wisdom to grayed hair (Van Der Geest, 2002). Among the Ga tribe in Southern Ghana, there is a common adage that underscores the value of old age that translates as: "the aged person is wiser than a sooth-sayer." Traditional, communal, and family-level authority is typically in the bosom of the aged in most Ghanaian communities. Thus, in decision-making, the aged are often accorded the honor of leadership (Dosu, 2014).

Throughout Ghana, children and young adults are trained to give up their seat for the aged. As a sign of respect, it is expected of young people to exchange respectful greetings with the aged and to offer to carry their loads when necessary. The aged are also traditionally considered to be the custodians of wisdom. These actions constitute a diverse but related system of beliefs, norms, values, and practices about old age that have been passed down from one generation to another, creating a mechanism by which younger members of society learn to venerate and cherish the need to support and provide for the aged in society. Notwithstanding these norms, the aged are expected to and do engage in activities such as fostering their grandchildren (Atobrah, 2016).

In addition to the above, specific traditional values and cultural prac-tices related to aging in Ghana are important. First, the hierarchical systems associated with wealth acquisition, custodianship of land, and other family property favor the aged. This is because the aged are revered as a source of wisdom. They are thus consulted for counseling and arbit-ration when conflicts arise. Moreover, they are deemed to be closer to the ancestors and thus they are expected to live honorably (including caring for their own children) so that they will "become" ancestors. This percep-tion is linked to an expectation of reciprocity of care; it means that chil-dren who have been cared for by their parents are obliged to provide care for their parents in their old age. A failure of this social contract on either side is thought to lead to adverse consequences.

The practice of reciprocity in parent–child relationship and other social relations ensures that resources flow from parents to children and subse-quently back from children to parents in their old age. This relationship often applies to persons who are biologically related as well as to situations of foster care. According to an Akan adage, often used as an admonition for children, "parents must care for children to grow their teeth and chil-dren must take care of their parents to lose theirs" (Apt, 1993). This cultural expectation serves to achieve two complementing benefits: it promotes a culture in which on one hand, child neglect is scorned and on the other hand care for the aged is appreciated. Moreover, it is believed that the wellbeing of the entire family can be affected by the neglect of care for any family member, including the aged. This belief is reinforced by the fear that able-bodied members of the family will incur the consequences of ancestral curses, if they failed in their duty to provide care for the aged.

Living arrangements of kin members favors inter-generational co-residence. Oppong's (1975) study in Dagbon (in Northern Ghana) indi-cated that up to five generations co-reside in one household (Oppong, 1975). The large number of household members serves as resource pool from which support for the aged is drawn. Over time, however, co-residence of children and the aged parents has declined by progressive nucleation of the family, and limited space in households, particularly, in urban areas. As a result, a research in the Ashanti Region reported that among the aged studied, most of them (78 percent) lived either in a rented apartment or in a family house (Anning, 2012). More recently it has been reported that the aged in Ghana are living in two generation households (WHO, 2014). This change in living arrangements has implications for the aged for accessing care. About 20 percent of the aged in Ghana usually live in small-size households that include one or two other household members (GSS, 2013). Within these settings the aged persons (80 years and above), who are often frail and in need of support for activities for daily living, lack access to support to deal with physical and emotional challenges, including effects of social distance and loneliness.

This change in living situation has also been influenced by factors such as occupational demands that make co-residence of parents and children and the aged more challenging (D. M. Badasu, 2004, 2012). There are also gender differences. Aged men in Ghana are more likely to live in nuclear households. Aged women on the other hand are likely to live in extended family households (Mba, 2010) and in most cases providing support for their offspring or other family members as caregivers for grandchildren (biological or non-biological).

Culturally defined status regarding the aged also exists and differs across Ghanaian society. It may not be based on chronological age. Therefore, greater emphasis is laid on the social functions performed by persons deter-mined as elderly. Persons performing certain functions are therefore ascribed the status of elderly persons irrespective of their chronological age. In African societies, for example, the role of grand-mother or grand-father may be performed by persons in their 30s or 40s if these have chil-dren who have started child-bearing at early or teenage years. Despite the relatively young age of the grandparents, they are considered as elders in society. Among some Ghanaian ethnic groups (for example Ewe and Kasena), any mother whose children have started bearing children is expected to stop bearing children and provide care for her grandchildren.

She is considered to have attained "social menopause" (Atobrah, 2016; Awedoba, 2002). Consequently, attaining the position of an elderly person in reproductive matters such as menopause is culturally determined.

Modernization, changing lifestyle, occupation demands, and social life have been undermining the values associated with care for the aged (Aboh & Ncama, 2017; Dosu, 2014; Tawiah, 2011). Migration and urbanization have reduced access to kin group members' assistance; geographic proximity is affected as younger members of the kin group work further away from home. Even when young parents live in the same city as their old parents, easy access that will enable care is affected by barriers such as vehicular traffic (D. M. Badasu, 2012). Further, the transportation system and associated infrastructure are not user-friendly for the aged (WHO, 2014). Thus, they may be inhibited by transportation even if they wanted to travel to visit their kin, as similarly observed elsewhere in Nigeria (GSS & United Nations Population Fund, 2013; Odufuwa, 2006). Demanding occupations put constrains on time needed by adult children to also care for their parents. The strain is especially severe in urban areas where work demands may be prioritized over social relationships.

Individualism has also weakened family ties. It has contributed to dependency on contemporary networks of social relations that include not only relatives but also friends and associated relations who provide financial and other forms of support for the aged. Some of these networks are found in churches, mosques, and other faith facilities. Hometown and old student associations have also been major sources of social capital for the aged (Tawiah, 2011).

Gendered experiences of aging in Ghana

The trend in growth of the aged population also shows that since 1984, a higher proportion of aged women than men are surviving beyond 60 years (Figure 5.2). Not only are more women living past the age of 60, they are also living longer than men, particularly beyond 75 years. This phenomenon has implications for designing interventions that meet the needs of aged women. As in other African countries, there are differences in economic and reproductive activity experiences of the male and female aged persons in Ghana (Aikins & Apt, 2016). Compared to males, female Ghanaians are more likely to work in the informal private sector and also more likely to continue working beyond 60 years. Moreover, elderly women often combine their economic activity with social reproduction activities such as performing childcare tasks, and caring for the sick. Younger women expect the support of their mothers for caring for their infants.

In traditional settings in Ghana, the practice whereby young women leave their matrimonial homes to go and live with their mothers or other older female kin until they have delivered and their child is a few months old before they return to their husband/partner enabled elderly women to contribute to social reproduction. Although this practice has declined because of urbanization, it places a demand on older women to meet the care needs of younger members of their kin while at the same time provided the needed help that they also may have.

On the other hand, men are particularly dependent on women for much of their needs including obtaining water, cooking and serving meals, laundry, and housekeeping, as part of traditional Ghanaian culture (Biritwum, Mensah, Yawson, & Minicuci, 2013). This expectation placed on women does not cease at advanced ages. Thus, even in a household of two that includes aged male and female persons, the women are more likely to serve the men and carry a greater burden of household chores. Outside of farming areas, this creates a situation where men's opportunity for physical activity is acutely limited.

Alternative care for the aged

As a result of changing living arrangements, families who can afford it are increasingly relying on hired non-family caregivers and care facilities for meeting the care needs of their aged. As the industry for such services in Ghana develops, it is transitioning gradually from informal to a more formal enterprise as some aged care agencies train their care providers prior to job placement (Coe, 2016). Commercial nursing agencies have emerged as a source of alternative and specialized care provision for the aged. These changes have some implications for the wellbeing of the aged. In particular, emotional care *may* not be ensured from a paid care giver (Coe, 2016).

In the last two decades, there has been increasing availability and access to public health care facilities and services for the aged, particularly those, who have terminal illnesses, chronic diseases such as renal failure, cancer, Type 2 diabetes, and hypertension. Routine screening for hypertension and other health conditions are provided in some care facilities. Also, some employers, and corporate organizations offer health-screening services to employees and focus on conditions such as prostate, breast, and cervical cancers, and diabetes. Despite the promotion of these preventive health strategies, there is inadequate health personnel who are adequately equipped to provide targeted services for the aged.

Women are typically the primary providers of care for families, and are more likely to provide care for the aged. They are, therefore, secondary beneficiaries of alternative care. Thus, in situations where alternative care for the aged is not available, additional strain is placed on women, including elderly women in the home who typically assume the role care givers, in addition to other roles such as fulltime work, care for young children, among others (D. M. Badasu, 2012). In the urban Ghanaian context, it has been reported, recently, that the cost of care for one aged person per month is almost $200, plus the additional reported high burden of care (Nortey, Aryeetey, Aikins, Amendah, & Nonvignon, 2017).

Commercial caregiving for the aged is developing out of necessity and as a response to socio-cultural transformations. Culture is dynamic and so are the care practices that have been culturally determined. Generally, health care infrastructure for the aged, such as hospice care facilities, are available to only a few in urban centers.

Physical activity among the aged in Ghana

Within the general Ghanaian population, physically active lifestyles associated with being largely an agrarian society is gradually giving way to more sedentary behaviors as domestic activities, work, and transportation are influenced by technology and urbanization. This behavior transition partly explains the low level of physical activity reported by the various Demographic and Health Surveys since 2008. It is reported that only half of males and less than one-third of females aged 15–49 years engaged in vigorous physical activity lasting at least 15 minutes for 3 or more days in a week (GSS, GHS, & ICF International, 2015).

Among older persons aged 50 years and over, the estimated prevalence of high intensity physical activity was 63 percent (WHO, 2014). Nevertheless, those living in rural areas continue to be resilient; 74 percent of rural dwellers are active compared to 46 percent of urban dwellers. A sedentary lifestyle among the aged increases their risk or severity of NCDs, and injuries due to falls.

While the tradition of respect and veneration for the aged has a positive benefit in terms of providing a groundswell of support, it also has the potential unintended effect of keeping the aged away from engaging in physically tasking activities. For example, it is common practice for the aged to "sit in state" and superintend over social activities (like naming ceremonies, weddings, and funerals) while younger persons speak for and run errands on behalf of the aged. Also, increasing migration sometimes makes it difficult for the aged to take a journey for long distances to participate in social events held away from their communities.

In Ghana, most aged persons are likely to have worked in the private informal sector (mainly in agriculture) and, as a result, do not have a formal retirement arrangement. Such aged people continue to be active and work until they are incapable of doing so anymore. In rural areas where younger and stronger members of the population leave to find greener pastures in urban centers, the aged who continue to tend their farms have opportunity to engage in physical activity, unlike those living in urban areas.

On the other hand, those whose youthful days were spent working in formal employment often experience sudden onset of inactivity upon retirement at 60 years. Typically, migrants tend to return to rural communities when they retire from employment as a coping mechanism for high cost of urban living (Mba, 2010). It is not known how retiring to a rural community affects the physical activity behavior of the aged in Ghana. Another key aspect of physical activity among the aged is the built environment. Generally, open spaces are lacking in most urban residential areas. This is the result of a combination of poor city planning, unauthorized development, and rapid urbanization with the development of slums or overcrowded neighborhoods. According to a 2008 data sheet published by the African Population and Health Research Centre (APHRC), between 40 percent to over 90 percent of urban populations in Sub-Saharan African countries live in slums. The built environment in such places is congested and prevents residents from engaging in physical activity.

There are currently no guidelines for Ghanaians on how to live a physically active lifestyle, and specifically, the aged. This lack of policy environment creates a dearth of motivation for the aged to be physically active. This is particularly important in urban areas where opportunities for physical activity is limited (Aryeetey, 2011; Tuakli-Wosornu, Rowan, & Gittelsohn, 2014).

Recommendations for an aging-friendly Ghana

Addressing issues of the aged in Ghana requires concerted action and working of multiple sectors in a coordinated fashion. But first, the actions should be guided by policy. In Ghana, there is no shortage of relevant policies to address the challenges of older persons. For example, there is a National Aging Policy (2010), and it aptly addresses issues related to the rights of the aged as well as their access to social, health and other services (Government of Ghana, 2010). The policy provides strategies for addressing social exclusion, health, social services, and general wellbeing among the aged. It also emphasizes cross-cutting issues relating to empowering families and communities, improving income security and enhanced social welfare for older persons. The exemption policy for the aged (70 years and older) by the NHIS eliminates financial barriers to access to health care (MOH, 2004). The exemption policy, however, needs to overcome the challenges of identifying the poor (D. Badasu, 2001). Further, a national social protection policy also targets the aged as a key vulnerable group through multiple actions including cash transfers, pension, and others (Government of Ghana, 2015). These and other policies demonstrate government's political will toward the welfare of the aged.

Ghana has also placed its human development goals and agenda within the broader Sustainable Development Goals (SDGs) and the long-term development agenda of the African Union (AU), known as Agenda 2063 (African Union Commission, 2015; United Nations Development

Program, 2016). The main guiding principles of the SDGs and the Agenda 2063 are inclusive and equitable sustainable development with emphasis on human development. Beyond the documented political will, there is need for investment in the policies as well as coordination of actions across the multiple agencies involved in the implementation of aging policies, strategies, and programs.

Regarding the promotion of an active lifestyle, it is important to situate interventions within the cultural context of Ghana. As indicated earlier, reciprocity is a core tenet of Ghanaian culture. Thus, promoting interventions that link the lifestyle of the aged with their offspring is likely to yield positive results. Such interventions can be integrated into efforts of preparing adults for aging, part of which involves encouraging adults to invest in the care of their own children as well as non-biological children who can then support them in their old age. The current situation in which many children are neglected suggests that the parents who neglect these children are likely to be neglected in their old age. This cycle can be broken when cultural values such as reciprocity are integrated into human development strategies.

It has been argued that a culturally relevant retirement policy is what Ghana needs for its retirees and the aged. For example, in the Ghanaian context, retiring without ownership of a home can affect quality of life economically and emotionally. Today, some older persons are retiring without any home of their own and with no hope for living their retirement in dignity, under such conditions the aged lose respect from the extended family and others. Another important dimension is the need to increase coverage of pension schemes to include the majority of Ghanaians who work in the informal sector and thus lack the benefits that a retired person can get with a pension.

Policies addressing the physical activity status of the aged will have to be designed to be disability-friendly and also encourage those who are not working to engage in some physical activity. The gender differences are also important. Therefore, policies addressing physical inactivity among the aged will have to consider the gender dimensions as well.

Loss of physical activity from social engagements can be replaced by volunteering activities. Club activities can be promoted among the aged to keep them active and provide them with opportunities for interaction, as it is currently being done by the Association of Ghana's Elders (AGE). All these suggestions can reduce social exclusion among the aged and prevent the negative effects of the socio-cultural transformation that affect the status of the aged and threatens their social engagement. Social engagement of the aged also removes the labeling of them as dependent and provides opportunities to be socially reintegrated into society.

Conclusion

The aged in Ghana is a growing population. They often live with NCDs, disability, and, less commonly, abuse from caregivers. They are often poor, and those in rural areas are likely to keep working through retirement age, until their bodies give up. Most of the aged in Ghana live in rural areas, but there is evidence of greater unmet need for services in urban areas. Although their needs are recognized at the highest political levels, there is insufficient investment in programs to meet the needs of the aged. Aging in Ghana is interwoven into its specific cultural and traditional fabric that is less often conducive to meeting the needs of women. These traditions supported elderly care in traditional settings in the past but are breaking down with the emergence of modern lifestyles that characterize urbanization and emerging technologies. Policies have been established, but detailed programs and specific investments are needed to promote active living of the elderly in Ghana, including physical activity guidelines, appropriate programs, and qualified providers.

References

Aboh, I. K. & Ncama, B. P. (2017). Critical Review of the Plight of the Ghanaian Aged. *IOSR Journal of Nursing and Health Science, 6*(2), 1–4. doi:10.9790/1959-0602070104.

African Union Commission. (2015). *Agenda 2063. The Africa We Want*. Addis Ababa: African Union Commission. Retrieved from www.un.org/en/africa/osaa/pdf/au/agenda2063.pdf.

Aikins, A. d.-G. & Apt, N. A. (2016). Aging in Ghana: Setting Priorities for Research, Intervention and Policy. *Ghana Studies, 19*(1), 35–45. doi:10.1353/ghs.2016.0002.

Anning, A. (2012). *The Emerging Problems of the Aged in Ghana: Issues of Housing And Basic Care: A Case Study of some Selected Districts in Ashanti Region*. (Master of Science), Kwame Nkrumah University of Science and Technology, Kumasi.

Apt, N. A. (1993). Care of the Elderly in Ghana: An Emerging Issue. *Journal of Cross-Cultural Gerontoly, 8*(4), 301–312. doi:10.1007/bf00972559.

Aryeetey, R. (2011). Environmental Barriers to Physical Activity in East Legon: A Qualitative Street Audit. *Ghana Physical Education and Sports Journal, 2*(2), 42–50.

Aryeetey, R., Aikins, M., Dako-Gyeke, P., & Adongo, P. (2015). Pathways Utilized for Antenatal Health Seeking among Women in the Ga East District, Ghana. *Ghana Medical Journal, 49*(1), 44–49. doi:10.4314/gmj.v49i1.8

Atobrah, D. (2016). Elderly Women, Community Participation and Family Care in Ghana: Lessons from HIV Response and AIDS Orphan Care in Manya Krobo. *Ghana Studies, 19*(1), 73–94.

Awedoba, A. K. (2002). Kassena Norms and Reproductive Health. *Institute of Africa Studies Research Review, 18*(1), 13–26.

Ayernor, P. K. (2012). Diseases of Ageing in Ghana. *Ghana Medical Journal, 46*(2 Suppl.), 18–22.

Badasu, D. (2001). Public versus Private Resources for Management of Childbirth and Care. *Institute of African Studies Research Review, 17*(2), 45–61.

Badasu, D. M. (2004). Child Care among Ewe Migrants in Accra: Cases of Crisis. *Research Review, Supp 16*, 17–37.

Badasu, D. M. (Ed.) (2012). *Maternal Education, Child Care and Wellbeing Among Accra Migrants*. Bergen: BRIC.

Biritwum, R., Mensah, G., Yawson, A., & Minicuci, N. (2013). *Study on Global AGEing and Adult Health (SAGE) Wave 1: The Ghana National Report*. Geneva: World Health Organization. Retrieved from apps.who.int/healthinfo/systems/surveydata/index.php/catalog/6/download/1940.

Coe, C. (2016). Not a Nurse, Not a Househelp. *Ghana Studies, 19*(1), 46–72.

Dake, F. A., Tawiah, E. O., & Badasu, D. M. (2011). Sociodemographic Correlates of Obesity among Ghanaian Women. *Public Health Nutrition, 14*(7), 1285–1291. doi:10.1017/s1368980010002879.

de-Graft Aikins, A. (2007). Ghana's Neglected Chronic Disease Epidemic: A Developmental Challenge. *Ghana Medical Journal, 41*(4), 154–159.

de-Graft Aikins, A., Unwin, N., Agyemang, C., Allotey, P., Campbell, C., & Arhinful, D. (2010). Tackling Africa's Chronic Disease Burden: From the Local to the Global. *Global Health, 6*(5). doi:10.1186/1744-8603-6-5.

Dosu, G. (2014). *Elderly Care in Ghana*. London: HKAG Publications.

Duku, S. K., van Dullemen, C. E., & Fenenga, C. (2015). Does Health Insurance Premium Exemption Policy for Older People Increase Access to Health Care? Evidence from Ghana. *Journal of Aging Society Policy, 27*(4), 331–347. doi:10.1080/08959420.2015.1056650.

Ghana Statistical Service (GSS). (2013). *2010 Population and Housing Survey: National Analytical report*. Accra: Ghana Statistical Service. Retrieved from www.statsghana.gov.gh/docfiles/publications/2010_PHC_National_Analytical_Report.pdf.

Ghana Statistical Service (GSS), Ghana Health Service (GHS), & ICF International. (2015). *Demographic and Health Survey 2014*. Rockville, MD: GSS, GHS, ICF International.

Ghana Statistical Service & United Nations Population Fund. (2013). *2010 Population & Housing Census Report: The Elderly in Ghana*. Accra: Ghana Statistical Service, Republic of Ghana, and United Nations Population Fund (UNFPA). Retrieved from www.statsghana.gov.gh/docfiles/publications/2010phc_the_elderly_in_Gh.pdf.

Government of Ghana. (2010). *National Aging Policy*. Accra: Ministry of Employment and Social Welfare. Retrieved from https://s3.amazonaws.com/ndpc-static/publication/Ageing+Policy_July+2010.pdf.

Government of Ghana. (2015). *Ghana National Social Protection Policy*. Accra: Ministry of Gender, Children, and Social Protection. Retrieved from www.social-protection.org/gimi/gess/RessourcePDF.action;jsessionid=5s0lYByW5h6Fyslp0nn vmQdyTcKWKpwNpc25dWwLcqJNhkxHD6ln!79209976?ressource.ressource Id=54058.

Mba, C. J. (2010). Population Ageing in Ghana: Research Gaps and the Way Forward. *Journal of Aging Research*, 1–8 . doi:10.4061/2010/672157.

Ministry of Health (MOH). (2004). *National Health Insurance Policy Framework for Ghana*. Accra, Ghana: MOH.

Nortey, S. T., Aryeetey, G. C., Aikins, M., Amendah, D., & Nonvignon, J. (2017). Economic Burden of Family Caregiving for Elderly Population in Southern Ghana: The Case of a Peri-urban District. *International Journal for Equity in Health, 16*(1), 16. doi:10.1186/s12939-016-0511-9.

Odufuwa, O. B. (2006). Enhancing Mobility of the Elderly in Sun-Saharan African Cities through Improved Public Transportation. *IATSS Research, 30*(1), 60–66.

Oppong, C. (1975). *Growing up in Dagbon*. Accra: Ghana Publishing Corporation.

Population Reference Bureau. (2016). *2016 World Population Data Sheet*. Population Reference Bureau. Retrieved from www.prb.org/pdf16/prb-wpds2016-web-2016.pdf.

Stewart Williams, J., Kowal, P., Hestekin, H., O'Driscoll, T., Peltzer, K., Yawson, A., Biritwum, R., Maximova, T., Salinas Rodriguez, A., Espinoza, B. M., Wu, F., Arokiasamy, P., Chatterji, S., & SAGE collaborators. (2015). Prevalence, Risk Factors and Disability Associated with Fall-related Injury in Older Adults in Low- and Middle-income Countries: Results from the WHO Study on Global AGEing and Adult Health (SAGE). *BMC Medicine, 13*(1), 147. doi:10.1186/s12916-015-0390-8.

Tawiah, E. O. (2011). Population Aging in Ghana: A Profile and Emerging Issues. *African Population Studies, 25*(2), 623–645.

The World Bank. (2017). Ghana. Retrieved from http://data.worldbank.org/country/ghana.

Tuakli-Wosornu, Y. A., Rowan, M., & Gittelsohn, J. (2014). Perceptions of Physical Activity, Activity Preferences and Health among a Group of Adult Women in Urban Ghana: A Pilot Study. *Ghana Medical Journal, 48*(1), 3–13.

United Nations Development Program. (2016). *Sustainable Development Goals*. New York: United Nations Development Program. Retrieved from www.undp.org/content/dam/undp/library/corporate/brochure/SDGs_Booklet_Web_En.pdf.

United Nations Population Fund (UNFPA). (2016). *State of the World's Population 2016*. New York: UNFPA. Retrieved from www.unfpa.org/sites/default/files/pub-pdf/The_State_of_World_Population_2016_-_English.pdf.

Van Der Geest, S. (2002). Respect and Reciprocity: Care of Elderly People in Rural Ghana. *Journal of Cross-Cultural Gerontology, 17*(1), 3–31.

World Health Organization (WHO). (2014). *Ghana Country Assessment Report on Ageing and Health*. Switzerland: WHO.

Part II

Effects of physical activity and exercise on the aging population

Chapter 6

Aging and health promotion in Brazil

Maria Beatriz Rocha Ferreira,
Antonia Dalla Pria Bankoff, and
Eliana Lucia Ferreira

Introduction

The aging process is a global phenomenon that deserves special attention in our society. The perception of aging is changing with the course of social development and it has to be understood in its history. The perception of aging depends on time and the state of society, and it is group specific. How to treat and care for the older adults is an aspect specific to socialization of human beings and changes of power in society.

The sociologist Nobert Elias (2001, 7) says

> life in actual societies has become more predictable, while demanding from each individual a higher degree of foresight and control of the passions. The relatively high life expectancy of individuals in these societies is a reflection of the increased security. [...] The prevention and treatment of illness in the present century are better organized than ever before, inadequate as they may still be. The internal pacification of society, the individual's protection against violence not sanctioned by the state, as against starvation, has reached a peak unimaginable to people of earlier times.

Today's perception of the elderly is the result of a long historical development, and actions come as result of the changes in the human interdependence network. Aging is considered a triumph of development. Increasing longevity is one of humanity's greatest achievements. People live longer because of improved nutrition, sanitation, medical advances, health care, education, and economic well-being according to the United Nations Population Fund (UNFPA, 2012, 16). This chapter presents the international and national documents that have influenced the development of the Brazilian public policies and civil societies programs, the demographic data, as well as the benefits of physical activity and programs for older adults in different parts of Brazil.

The international conferences and documents that influenced the Brazilian public policies were the *First World Assembly on Aging* held in Vienna in 1982 and the *Second World Assembly on Aging* held in Madrid in 2002 (UN, 2002, 16) and later, the document of *Aging in the Twenty-first Century: A Celebration and a Challenge* (UNFPA, 2012). These documents were the base for the development of the international human rights instruments and their translation into national laws and regulations, and influenced the affirmative measures in the country. International agreements were significant for the development of the public policies, but also the initiatives of civil societies, scientific exchanges, social movements (non-governmental organizations—NGOs) and the social networks in Brazil (through media) were fundamental for the social development for older adults.

The Constitution of the Federative Republic of Brazil in 1988 was an important landmark in health, education, and human rights. Public health policies were elaborated with the purpose of drawing attention to the entire population, through actions to promote, protect, and recover health, guaranteeing integration of care. That includes meeting the different realities and health needs of the population and individuals. The Unified Health System (SUS—Sistema Único de Saúde) was created as an important goal to attend, especially for the low social class population (BRASIL, 2010, 19).

Faced with the growing demands of an aging population and in accordance with the rights provided for in the 1988 Constitution, in 1994 the National Policy for the Elderly was promulgated through Law 8.842/94, regulated in 1996 by Decree 1948/96. This policy guarantees social rights to older adults, creating conditions to promote their autonomy, integration, and effective participation in society and reaffirming their right to health in the different levels of care of the Unified Health System. In 1999, The National Policy for the Elderly was established and, in 2002, the organization and implementation of the State Health Care Networks for the Elderly was proposed (BRASIL, 2010, 19).

In 2003, the National Congress approved and the President of the Republic sanctioned the Statute of the Elderly, which is considered one of the greatest social achievements of the older population in our Brazil, broadening the response of the State and society to the needs of this population (BRASIL, 2010, 17–19). In the sport and leisure arena, this proposal led to the establishment of partnerships for the implementation of programs of physical and recreational activities for older adults (BRASIL, 2010, 31).

In 2006, the Ministry of Health updated the National Health Policy for the Elderly and focused on a new paradigm, including the various functional capacities when formulating policies for the health of the elderly population. This improved law takes into consideration that there are older people, quite independent, and another portion of the population more fragile; thus, actions should be based on these specificities. In addition, the promotion of Active and Healthy Aging, in accordance with the recommendations of the United Nations (Madrid Plan 2002) is part of the policy guidelines. The fundamentals of the policy are (a) active participation of older adults in society and in the development, and the fight against poverty; (b) promotion of health and well-being in old age: promotion of healthy aging; (c) supportive environment conducive to aging, and (d) promotion of socio-educational and health resources directed to older adults (BRASIL, 2010, 23).

The demographic data gives significant information for the development of public health in all age categories of the population. According to the most recent projection of the population, carried out by the Brazilian Institute of Geography and Statistics (IBGE), the group of older people aged 60 years and older will increase from 13.8 percent in 2020 to 33.7 percent in 2060, which marks it an increase of 20 percent. The group of older people aged 60 years and older will be higher than the group of children up to 14 years of age after 2030, and in 2055, the participation of older adults in the total population will be greater than that of children and youngsters up to 29 years of age (IBGE, 2013).

The 2010 demographic data point out the varying need of improvement in different sectors of the Brazilian society, focusing on the greater longevity of people. Between 2002 and 2012, Brazil underwent changes that produced significant impacts on the living conditions of the population, such as dynamics in the labor market; rights and benefits linked to the human rights; valuation of the minimum wage; creation, expansion, and consolidation of a set of public policies related to work; health and education; as well as improvement of living conditions and well-being, such as adequate sanitation, health programs, incidence control of various diseases, among others (IBGE, 2013). As a result of these factors, the epidemiological transition characterized a change in the morbidity and mortality profile of the population, with a progressive decrease in deaths due to infectious diseases and an increase in deaths due to chronic diseases. This fact provoked a need for the country to adapt an entire system that treats children with infectious parasitic diseases as a priority over older people suffering from chronic degenerative diseases. This paradigm shift was instrumental in thinking about health and education programs starting at a young age in order to prevent future problems. These changes are still an ongoing process (BRASIL, 2010). Today there are three programs in particular that receive specific funds: care for the elderly, hypertensitivity, and women. This was a breakthrough for the elderly.

Physical activity benefits

The World Health Organization (WHO) has established many documents supporting the development of physical activity (WHO, 2002, 2004).

Healthy and active aging is a challenge in today's world. The definition of active aging is

> the process of optimizing opportunities for health, participation and security in order to enhance quality of life as people age. [...] The word "active" "refers to continuing participation in social, economic, cultural, spiritual and civic affairs, not just the ability to be physically active or to participate in the labor force.
>
> (WHO, 2002, 12)

The document calls attention to how the participation in regular, moderate physical activity can delay functional declines, reduce the onset diseases in both healthy and chronically ill people, and reduce the severity of disabilities associated with heart disease and brain stroke. Besides these positive influences, older adults can improve their mental health, social contacts, and reduce risk of falls and medical costs, among others (WHO, 2002, 23).

The global recommendations on physical activity for health (WHO, 2010) established levels of physical activity for population, recommendations to increase physical activity, and policies to address insufficient physical activity. For older adults physical activity includes: recreational or leisure-type physical activity, transportation (e.g., walking or cycling), occupational (if the person is still engaged in work), household chores, plays, games, sports or organized physical activity, and functional exercise related to daily life, family, and community activities. Any physical activity will improve cardiorespiratory and muscular fitness, bone and functional health, and reduce the risk of non-communicable diseases (NCDs), depression, and cognitive decline.

Alves, Leite, and Machado (2008) emphasize the importance of functional capacity in older age. Maintaining all the functions translates into fewer problems for the individual, family, or society. Problems start when the functions begin to deteriorate and the person becomes dependent (Alves, Leite, & Machado, 2008). These authors also consider the gender issue, since a greater prevalence of frailty in women can be explained by the greater physiological loss of female muscle mass with aging. In addition, women seem to be more prone to the development of sarcopenia, which is a risk intrinsic to the development of the syndrome. Other hypotheses are based on the fact that women have higher survival rates and a higher prevalence of morbidities when compared with men, who have a higher mortality rate for the same age (Alves, Leite, & Machado, 2008).

Studies were carried out in Brazil on functional disability and health profiles of older adults, as well as their prevalence rates, based on the National Household Sample Survey for 2003. The sample size was 33,786 older individuals. The results showed that the health of the older population can be described through three profiles: (1) *healthy older adult*—with a lower probability of disability and chronic illness, and more active group, those who practice physical activity; (2) *older adult with mild functional disability*—with mainly hypertension and lower back problems, who were still independent in activities of daily living, although with high difficulty in mobility; and (3) *older adult with severe functional disability*—with higher probability of chronic illness, high difficulty with activities of daily living, and high dependency in terms of mobility. The greatest difference observed between these three groups was attributed to "functional capacity." Thus, functional capacity is the major determinant of health profiles of older adults in Brazil, rather than the presence of disease (Alves, Leite, & Machado, 2008).

Research further shows that aging also reduces the number of motor units. This phenomenon appears to be a result of loss of alpha motor neurons from the spinal cord with subsequent degeneration of its neurons in contrast to the remaining motor units increasing in size. In addition, it is denoted in the aged reduced capacity to generate force in high speed (power). Several studies have related the reduction of muscular strength to a greater susceptibility to falls, fractures, and dependence of older people. The reduction of aerobic capacity in older adults has been attributed to their loss of muscle mass (Spirduso, Francis, & MacRae, 2005).

Epidemiological studies in different countries have confirmed the decisive role of physical activity in promoting health, quality of life, and prevention and control of various diseases. Guidelines for the promotion of healthy lifestyles have been recommended by organizations involved with public health, highlighting the practice of regular physical activity throughout the life cycle of the human being offered by governmental, nongovernmental, and scientific organizations (Bankoff & Jurado, 2013; Matsudo, Matsudo, & Marin, 2008; Pollock & Wilmore, 1993).

Matsudo, Matsudo, and Marim (2008) published a review on physical activity and healthy life. The level of physical conditioning in older adults is a predictor of mortality and does not depend on abdominal or total adiposity. Recent studies highlight the positive impact of regular physical activity on cognitive aspects, mental health, and overall well-being of the individual during the aging process. Some highlight the effect of physical activity, more specifically walking, which reduces the risk of vascular dementia, among others, as well as the existence of less cognitive decline in those with healthy habits.

Bankoff and Jurado (2013) emphasize that the benefits of exercising regularly are beneficial to all organs in an aging body, especially in the areas of cardiorespiratory, locomotor, digestive, and renal functions. It is common for older adults to take various types of medications, especially for blood pressure, causing various side effects, such as constipation. In this case, physical exercise is an important adjuvant for bowel functions. Another finding in this research was that older adults reported difficulties in swallowing during meals and a feeling of "suffocation" due to short breaths when swallowing. When breathing exercises and strengthening of the muscles involved in breathing were included in the exercise routine these difficulties disappeared.

The association between levels of physical activity and usage of medication in older women was studied by Silva, Azevedo, Matsudo, and Lopes (2012). The level of physical activity was assessed using a pedometer, and the use of medication was assessed through medical records supplied by the Family Health Programme in the city of São Caetano do Sul, State of São Paulo. Regular use of pharmaceuticals, regardless of type of illness or treatment, was listed. The results of the study indicated that, among the 271 women involved in the study, 84.9 percent had been classified as active. Only 23.2 percent did not use any type of medication, while 29.8 percent used three or more medications. The level of physical activity was inversely associated with the number of medications used. The study concluded that higher volumes of physical activity were significantly associated with lower usage of pharmaceuticals in women who are involved in a physical activity program.

Dissemination of the scientific knowledge

In Brazil, the information of the scientific research is centralized on websites of the federal government, universities, National Council of Scientific and Technological Development (CNPq, *SciELO Scientific Electronic Library Online—Citation Index online*), among others. In addition, the Brazilian government and civil societies work together to disseminate information about older adults. Programs are carried out in partnerships with the Public and Private Services, NGOs, and other institutions. The means of communication are diverse, including classes or web networks, blogs, Facebook, magazines, books, and distance learning. They constantly disseminate information on health, culture, longevity, and the benefits of physical activity in the aging process. For instance, the Movement and Health (Saúde Em Movimento, 2017) is a website that publishes information on aging and its relationships with physical activity. The website also emphasizes that regular physical exercise is recognized. This information is based on guidelines of the American College of Sports Medicine (ACSM), the Centres for Disease Control and Prevention (CDC), the Brazilian Society of Geriatrics, the Centre of Studies of the Physical Fitness Laboratory of São Caetano do Sul (CELAFISCS), and other scientific recognized organizations.

The Portal also emphasizes that regular physical exercise is recognized as the way to prevent and combat or prolong the occurrence of the illnesses associated with aging. If people engage in regular physical activity, their health should improve as well as their quality of life. Furthermore, benefits include: increase of autonomy and sense of well-being, improvement of cardiovascular conditioning, increase of muscular strength, maintenance or development of flexibility, coordination and balance, incentive to social contact and pleasure of life, weight and nutritional control, promotion of relaxation, reduction of anxiety, insomnia and depression, maintenance of libido and sexual vigor (Saúde Em Movimento, 2017). The Bulletin of the Health Institute (BIS) of the State Government of São Paulo is another way to release information to promote the debate on health based on qualified information, as well as contributing to decision-making in the formulation of public policies, based on a broad discussion of concepts and trends in the health field. Matsudo (2009) emphasizes the benefits of physical activity related to anthropometric characteristics, cognitive and psychosocial effects, metabolic effects, cognitive and psychosocial effects, effects on falls and therapeutic effect.

Governmental and non-governmental physical activity programs

Since 2003, the Ministry of Sports in Brazil has been developing the Sports and Leisure Programme in the City (PELC) with the following goals: to provide the practice of physical, cultural, and leisure activities that involve all age groups and adults with disabilities; to stimulate the social coexistence; and the training of managers and community leaders. This program further focuses on the research and socialization of knowledge and its contribution for sports and leisure to be treated as policies and rights for all. In 2012, the PELC Healthy Living for older adults was created (ME, 2017).

Brazilian public universities at the federal and state levels have three aims: graduate and undergraduate teaching, scientific research, and extension and outreach programs. Physical activity programs for older adults are included in the extension and outreach programs of public access. For example, the Programme of Coexistence and Social Inclusion on Physical Activity and Health (Mexa-se UNICAMP) of the State University of Campinas was created in 2004, in partnership with the Laboratory of Postural Evaluation (LAP) of the Faculty of Physical Education and the Centre of the Community (Cecom-Unicamp). It is part of the university's Institutional Quality of Life Project. The aims of this program are: to raise awareness and stimulate the university population about the practice of physical activities as a factor of health promotion and prevention of chronic noncommunicable diseases; to increase the level and regularity of the practice of physical activities, favoring the daily activities developed at Unicamp; to make the community of the State University of Campinas aware of the importance of physical activity for biopsychosocial well-being and improvement in the overall quality of life (Bankoff, Zamai, & Moraes, 2010).

Unicamp also offers the UniversIDADE Programme created in 2014 linking academic and popular education for adults 50+ providing the Community of Unicamp and city of Campinas with their pre-retirement, retirement, and post-retirement programs. The aims are to keep older people active, both physically and mentally, by considering the need for prevention, stimulation, and training of the physical and emotional development. These interdisciplinary activities seek to foster dialogues related to longevity and quality of life, including the following areas of knowledge: art and culture, sports and leisure, physical and mental health, and culture and income generation. This program intends to work with integrating these activities, so that the individuals can interact with each other in teams. This allows the facilitator to define the needs, solutions and execution for the individuals (Programa UniversIDADE, 2017).

The Physical Education program for Older Adults at the School of Physical Education and Sport at the University of São Paulo was created in 1994 aiming to improve and maintain the motor and functional abilities of older adults. It provides the undergraduate students with practical experiences within their academic training and serves as the basis for scientific research as well as the community outreach at the University of São Paulo (USP, 2017).

Another program was created in 1974. The Centre of Studies of the Physical Fitness Research Laboratory of São Caetano do Sul (CELAFISCS) is one of the most significant institutions in Sport Sciences in Latin America, which has received global recognition awards. They have developed various research projects, among them the Mixed Longitudinal Study on Active Elderly Adults of São Caetano do Sul (CELAFISCS, 2016). In 1966, CELAFISCS launched the "Agita São Paulo" Program (*agita* means to move the body) as an agreement with the State Department of Health of São Paulo, and partnerships that currently involve governmental and non-governmental institutions, as well as private companies. The aim is to combat sedentary lifestyles in the State of São Paulo by promoting physical activity and active lifestyles. The program's actions intend to reach the general population with three main target groups: students (Agita Galera), workers, and older adults. Their successes have reached different states in Brazil and various other countries in Latin America, and include the global *World Agita* program (Matsudo et al., 2003).

One focus of this program is the older population. The prescription for this population is to perform moderate physical activities for at least 30 minutes a day on most days of the week. The key of this new concept is that any activity of daily life is valid and that activities can be carried out continuously or at intervals. Thus, the most important thing is to accumulate about 30 minutes of activity per day (Matsudo et al., 2003). The diagnostic evaluation of the Agita São Paulo Program for older adults 50+ from small cities and metropolitan areas (São Caetano do Sul) in the State of São Paulo evaluated the level of knowledge, barriers, and facilitators to practice physical activity in a sample of more than 2,000 individuals (Matsudo, Matsudo, & Barros Neto, 2001). The barriers mentioned in the study include the lack of equipment and the need for rest are common in both regions; location, climate, and lack of skill are common barriers only for the cities in the countryside; while lack of time, knowledge, and fear of injury are barriers for the metropolitan area. Thus, the perceived barriers are not only related to the physical, but also depend on the will and motivation of the people. Unfortunately, despite the efforts to reduce the physical barriers in the physical activity programs of the different institutions, the majority of the population is still sedentary, which implies a public health problem.

Aging adults with disabilities

Aging adults with disabilities have recently been included in the discussion in the last decades, precisely because until recently most of the disabled adults did not experience this phase of life. The scientific and social advances have generally promoted an increase in the longevity of the population at large, including the longevity of adults with disabilities. According to De Queiroz Brito, De Oliveira, and Eulálio (2015), the aging of adults with disabilities brings several functional losses and a high rate of dementia, due to the prolonged use of medications causing secondary health problems, such as demineralization, osteoporosis, and movement disorders, inducing mobility and decrease in muscular strength. Generally, adults with disabilities start showing signs of aging from the age at 30+ or 40+, which implies the need for specific care.

In Brazil, older adults with disabilities have relevance in the field of human rights, public health, and the social and sporting domains (BRASIL, 2015). It is noteworthy that the situation of assistance for disabled older persons still presents a profile of fragility and discontinuity of actions in both the public and private sectors. This is related to the socio-cultural constructions of people with disabilities for thousands of years and the stigmatizing and exclusion they have received and are still experiencing from many parts of social life.

The research on disability in the 2010 Demographic Census was based on the individual's perception of their difficulty in seeing, hearing or getting around, and in the existence of mental or intellectual disability (IBGE, 2012). The adults with disabilities data show that they can benefit from more consistent outreach programs. Although there have been advances in terms of rights, established through legal institutes, there is still a long way between the legally established and the reality experienced. Several institutions in Brazil have developed physical activity programs involving all age groups, including older adults with disabilities aiming at social interaction, sport, leisure, and, above all, improvement in quality of life (Ferreira, 2010). Dancing in wheelchairs is one of the most recent artistic and sportive movements reaching all ages. It incorporates modern dance, ballroom dance, and therapeutic dance. Initially, the focus was the artistic and demonstrative execution, and since 1975, it has been organized as competitive wheelchair dance. This athletic dance has its own criteria and is inserted in a complex web loaded with cultural and sportive meanings. The Brazilian Confederation of Dance in Wheelchair has organized many events, as well as scientific congresses. More than 60 percent of these athletes are of advanced ages. The benefits of the research related to this Confederation points out the fact that different "bodies" are conquering new social spaces (Ferreira, 2010).

In Brazil, research centers of higher education institutions, such as the Nucleus of Research in Inclusion, Motion and Distance Learning at the Federal University of Juiz de Fora, Federal University of Uberlândia, Federal University of Minas Gerais, State University of Campinas, and the State University of São Paulo and others carry out research in partnership with Paralympic institutions. The purpose is the generation of knowledge about the demands of adults with disabilities, planning sports activities, as well as implementing clinical, therapeutic, and pedagogical strategies for institutions to develop programs that focus on all different ability levels with the aim to prevent losses and maintain the acquired skills.

Aging indigenous peoples

The aging indigenous peoples in Brazil have different experiences compared to urban adults. The total indigenous population in Brazil consists of 896,917 individuals, approximately 0.4 percent of the country's population, incorporating 305 ethnic groups and 192 languages. The 2010 census counted the number of indigenous peoples from the group of people who declared themselves or considered themselves indigenous, based on a community defined by linguistic, social and cultural affinity (IBGE, 2012). They are in different stages of organizations and locations. Their spatial distribution is the result of a historical process of socioeconomic occupation in Brazil, which has led to a cultural and territorial identity of this population throughout time (IBGE, 2012). Some indigenous people live in cities, some in reservations not too far from the cities, and others have very little contact with urban areas. Some indigenous people live in cities, some in reservations not too far from the cities, and others have very little contact with urban areas.

The ancestral indigenous education was transmitted from the parents and extended family in their communities. Each ethnical group has its own way to take care of children, youth, and older adults in Brazil. Despite differences in the social system and linguistic families of indigenous societies, the basis of the societal organization is similar. The extended families are the base of their social organization and the aging indigenous members have a special role in their systems. They hold knowledge and wisdom, and all the information and authority passes through them. Indigenous body practices and/or indigenous games (definition below) vary depending on the ethnic group. The common element is that the aging adults have a key social role in their societies. They are the memory of the community, and so they hold a lot of power. Despite the silence and sanctions imposed by processes of oppression (for example, colonization, government programs for indigenous peoples and globalization), many of the indigenous games are still alive in the memories of older adults and have remained significant, at least in some communities (Rocha Ferreira, Mizrahi, & Capettini, 2016).

> Traditional indigenous games are physical activities with recreational or playful features permeated by myths and cultural values. They therefore encompass the material and immaterial worlds of each ethnic group. The games require the learning of specific motor skills, strategies and/or luck. They are usually played ceremonially during rituals to please a supernatural being and/or to obtain fertility, rain, food, health, physical fitness, success in war or other needs and hopes. They also aim at preparing young members for adult life, including socialization, cooperation and the training of warriors. The games take place at determined times and places, according to rules freely accepted but absolutely binding, and there is usually no age limit for players. In addition, the games do not necessarily have winners or losers, and no awards except prestige are granted. Participation itself is full of meaning and affords experiences that are incorporated by the group and the individual.
> (Rocha Ferreira, Vinha, Tagliari, Fassheber, & Ugarte, 2005, 33)

These games should not be considered as something from the past that has been frozen, archived, and preserved simply for posterity. They are an integral part in the very processes of ongoing sociocultural changes. The Indigenous People's Games is a movement created in 1966 by two brothers, Marcos and Carlos, from the Terena ethnic group and sponsored by the Brazilian Government (Rocha Ferreira, 2014). The aim of these games is celebration and not competition. In these games, active older indigenous men and women from different ethnic groups play together and enjoy all the various moments and movements together. They are in the dances, tug of war, arrow activities, blowgun, bowling ball, art and craft, as well as supervising the young generation. Thus, the indigenous games provide a wonderful example how all generations can play together and stay healthy and fit together, no matter the age.

Final considerations

The population increase in Brazil has triggered profound changes in society. The Brazilian government has signed and sought to comply with international documents on the issue of older adults over the last 30 years. This includes legislation, food improvement, minimum wage, health services, and the building of awareness programs of the importance of physical activity for adults 60+, although much still needs to be accomplished. Information on this issue has been disseminated by public agencies, such as the Ministry of Health, Sports and States, and through NGOs and other institutes. Researchers and programs on physical activity of older adults are carried out in public, private universities, and research centers. The investigations involving adults with disabilities and the impact that physical activity has on them are recent and deserve greater care and attention. The indigenous population has been the target of attention by the Brazilian government.

The challenges of the next years are to increase the number and quality of heath care programs all over the country and to provide more information about the risk factors associated with the lack of physical activity. In addition, adequate facilities are needed to offer physical activity programs that aim to combat the sedentary life style, and which ultimately can lead to behavioral changes toward a healthy life style.

References

Alves, L.C., Leite, I.C., & Machado, C.J. (2008). Perfis de saúde dos idosos no Brasil: análise da Pesquisa Nacional por Amostra de Domicílios de 2003 utilizando o método Grade of Membership. *Caderno de Saúde Pública*, Rio de Janeiro, 24(3), 535–546.

Bankoff, A. & Jurado, S.R. (2013). Prevalência de hipertensão e obesidade em participantes de uma Universidade da Melhor Idade. In V.C. Lourenço., C. Ferreira da Palma, W. Diego de Almeida, & F.R. Teodoro dos Santos. (editors). *Universidade da Melhor Idade*. Três Lagoas, MS: UFMS.

Bankoff, A.D.P., Zamai, C.A., & Moraes, M.A.A. (2010). *Manual de atividade física: Um guia para a saúde – Acorda!!! É hora de se cuidar. Programmea Mexase*. Retrieved from: http://mexase.cecom.unicamp.br/images/manual-mexa-se.pdf.

BRASIL. (2005). Presidência da República. Secretaria Especial dos Direitos Humanos. *A Convenção sobre os Direitos das Pessoas com Deficiência*, Brasília. Retrieved from: www.planalto.gov.br/ccivil_03/_ato2007-2010/2009/decreto/d6949.htm.

BRASIL. (2010). Ministério da Saúde. *Atenção à saúde da pessoa idosa e envelhecimento*. Brasília, DF. Retrieved from: http://bvsms.saude.gov.br/bvs/publicacoes/atencao_saude_pessoa_idosa_envelhecimento_v12.pdf.

BRASIL. (2015). Presidência da República. Secretaria Especial dos Direitos Humanos. *Convenção sobre os Direitos das Pessoas com Deficiência*, Brasília. Retrieved from: /www.planalto.gov.br/ccivil_03/_ato2007-2010/2009/decreto/d6949.htm.

CELAFISCS. Centre of Studies of the Physical Fitness Laboratory of São Caetano do Sul. (2016). Retrieved from: http://celafiscs.org.br.

De Queiroz Brito, D.T., De Oliveira, A.R., & Eulálio, M. (2015). De ciência física e envelhecimento: estudo das representações sociais de idosos sob reabilitação psioterápica. *Avances en Psicología Latinoamericana 33*(1), 121–133. Retrieved from: www.scielo.org.co/pdf/apl/v33n1/v33n1a09.pdf/.

Elias, N. (2001). *The loneliness of the dying*. New York: Continuum.

Ferreira, E.L. (2010). *Esportes e atividades físicas inclusivas*. Niteroi: Intertexto, 01.

Instituto Brasileiro de Geografia e Estatística (IBGE). (2012). Censo demográfico 2010. *Características Gerais da população, religião e pessoas com deficiência*. Rio de Janeiro, IBGE. Censo demogr.

Instituto Brasileiro De Geografia E Estatística (IBGE). (2013). *Estudos e Pesquisas: Informação Demográfica e Socioeconômica. Sintese de indicadores sociais. Uma análise das condições de vida*, Rio de Janeiro, IBGE. Censo demogr.

Matsudo, S. (2009). Envelhecimento, atividade física e saúde. Envelhecimento e Saúde. *Boletin Instituto de Saúde do Estado de São Paulo*. BIS 47, Brasil.

Matsudo, S.M.M., Matsudo, V.K.R., Araújo, T.L., Andrade, D.R., Andrade, E.L., Oliveira, L.C., & Braggion, G.F. (2003). The Agita São Paulo Programme as a model for using physical activity. *American Journal of Public Health*, 14(4), 265–272.

Matsudo, S.M.M., Matsudo, V.K.R., & Barros Neto, T.L. (2001). Atividade física e envelhecimento: aspectos epidemiológicos. *Revista Brasileira de Medicina do Esporte*, (7)1, 2–13.

Mastudo, S.M., Matsudo, V.K.R., & Marin, R.V. (2008). Atividade Física e Envelhecimento Saudável. *Diagnóstico & Tratamento*, 13, 142–147.

Ministério do Esporte – PELC (ME). (2017). Retrieved from: www.esporte.gov.br/index.php.

Pollock, M.L. & Wilmore, J.H. (1993). *Exercícios na Saúde e na Doença*. Rio de Janeiro: Medsi, pp. 145–168.

Programa UnivesIDADE. (2017). Retrieved from: www.programa-universidade.unicamp.br.

Rocha Ferreira, M.B. (2014). Indigenous games: a struggle between past and present. *International Council of Sport Science and Physical Education*, (ICSSPE) 67, 48–54.

Rocha Ferreira, M.B., Mizrahi, E., & Capettini, S.M.F. (2016). Indigenous women, games and ethno-sport in Latin America. In: R.L. De D'Amico, T. Benn, & G. Pfister (Eds.) *Women and sport in Latin America*. 1st ed. New York: Routledge – Taylor & Francis, 10–33.

Rocha Ferreira. M.B., Vinha, M., Tagliari, I.A., Fassheber, J.R., & Ugarte, M.C.D. (2005). Traditional native Brazilian (Indian) games (pp. 33–34) *Atlas do Esporte no Brasil*. Rio de Janeiro: Shape Editora e Promoções.

Saúde em Movimento. Terceira Idade – *Envelhecimento e suas relações com a Atividade Física*. (2017). Retrieved from: www.saudemmovimento.com.br/conteudos/conteudo_frame.asp?cod_noticia=85.

Silva, L.J., Azevedo, M.R, Matsudo, S., & Lopes, G.S. (2012). Association between levels of physical activity and use of medication among older women. *Caderno de Saúde Pública*, 28(3), 463–471.

Spirduso, W., Francis, K., & MacRae, P. (2005). *Physical dimensions of aging.* Champaign, IL: Human Kinetics.

UNFPA. United Nations Population Fund (2012). *Ageing in the twenty-first century: a celebration and a challenge.* New York, and HelpAge International, London. Retrieved from: www.unfpa.org/sites/default/files/pub-pdf/Ageing%20 report.pdf.

United Nations (UN). (2002). *Political declaration and Madrid international plan of action on aging.* New York: United Nations. Available from: www.un.org/en/ events/pastevents/pdfs/Madrid_plan.pdf.

Universidade de São Paulo (USP). (2017). *Programmea educação física para idosos.* Escola de Educação Física da Universidade de São Paulo. Retrieved from: www. eefe.usp.br/?curso_comunitario/mostrar/id/8.

World Health Organization (WHO). (2002). *Active aging. A policy framework.* Madrid, Spain. Retrieved from: http://apps.who.int/iris/bitstream/10665/67215/1/ WHO_NMH_NPH_02.8.pdf.

World Health Organization (WHO). (2004). *Global strategy on diet, physical activity and health, 2004.* Retrieved from: www.who.int/dietphysicalactivity/ strategy/eb11344/strategy_english_web.pdf.

World Health Organization (WHO). (2010). *Global recommendations on physical activity for health.* Retrieved from: http://apps.who.int/iris/bitstream/10665/443 99/1/9789241599979_eng.pdf.

Chapter 7

Healthy aging in Cuba through physical activity

Marta Cañizares Hernández (translated by Urbano Ramiro Cañizares Hernández)

Introduction

People over the age of 60 are the fastest growing segment of society today all over the world. In the past, old age was associated with illness, weakness, and inability to work, as described by Orosa's involutionary theories (Orosa, 2001). However, nowadays, specialists recognize the special phase the elderly are going through, and the equally significant role that healthcare professionals such as medical doctors, psychologists, social workers, as well as family members, friends, and neighbors play in their lives. An understanding of the elderly includes being receptive to their needs in the aging process. It also involves giving them reassurance and confidence and providing them with more space for personal realization (Beutel, Glaesmer, Decker, Fischbeck, & Brahler, 2009; Woodman, Akehurst, Hardy, & Beattie, 2010; Henry, 1990).

The personality traits of an elderly person are characterized by a tendency toward diminished self-esteem, physical, mental, and aesthetic decline, as well as a changing role in society. At this stage of their lives, older adults begin to show some deterioration in their cognitive, affective, and motivational skills caused by a diminishing perceptual acuity. They also begin to show memory loss and other emotional manifestations such as depression, anguish, anxiety, and various fears related to this decline. These manifestations affect the behavior of the aging individual.

In this chapter, we will analyze the specific situation of aging adults in Cuba in regards to their involvement in physical activity as health promoter. Cuban practitioners have long been engaged in providing meaningful physical engagement of the elderly, for example, through the so-called *Circulos de abuelos* (Grandparents' Clubs). These interventions have proven to support the aging process in a meaningful way that promotes health and self-confidence. Another example of taking care of the elderly through physical activity in Cuba is the support provided to aging athletes, who have formerly competed on the top-level for their country. These programs serve as excellent examples in the promotion of healthy aging in Cuba.

Classification of the elderly

There are three classifications for defining the elderly person that were laid out by Fritz Giese at the X Congress on Psychology held in Bonn (cited by Tolstij, 1989). These classifications are namely, the *negativist*, the *extrovert*, and the *introvert*. Older people with a negativist view refuse to accept the existence of any sign of old age. The extrovert's view recognizes the arrival of old age in the reality of reaching retirement age as well as their clashing world views with the younger generation within their social and family lives. And the introvert looks at the person and their experiences as they progress in the aging process. These experiences include intellectual and emotional changes that are associated with the loss of relationships, new interest, reminiscences, diminished mobility, and the search for tranquility, among other changes.

This three-fold classification by Tolstij allows us to group older people under one type or another, so that their personality restructuring can be assessed in the actual context. These assessments, however, are always an approximation in the process of analysis of the manifestations of the aging process, but they can be helpful for scientists and practitioners working with older people.

Social role and caring for the elderly

There are many elderly people who, even though they are aware of the aging process they are going through, still have a proper assessment of their characteristics and their real possibilities, and they are willing to actively play their role in society (Daure, 2015). Tolstij (1989) stresses the active role that wisdom and experience play in the aging process, which he characterizes as a privilege enjoyed by mature and older people. This is not only the individual's recollection of the past, but also their ability to orient themselves quickly in the present by using both their personal experience as well as the experience learned or acquired from other people (Saavedra and Villalta, 2008). In today's Cuban society, great efforts are made to provide the elderly with social well-being, not only in a material sense, but also by helping them to participate actively in society to the best of their abilities.

The government has also taken measures to enable people who have reached retirement age to stay in their job if they wish to do so. This project has led to the creation of educational actions that are aimed at enriching the social and spiritual life of the elderly as well as how they take care of themselves. All of this contributes to the creation of a positive and healthy image of the overall aging process in humans. This approach prepares the family, especially the new generation, to live harmoniously with the older generation, which strengthens and develops activities in the community.

In our country, research studies regarding old age are conducted by El Centro Iberoamericano de la III Edad (CITED), which is the Iberian-American Center for Old Age, located at the Hospital Calixto Garcia in Havana City. This research center focuses on the training of human resources favoring a more comprehensive approach of the care of elderly people.

The Faculty of Psychology at the University of Havana has created a branch called Cátedra Universitaria del Adulto Mayor (University Center for Old Age Research), as well as the University for Elderly People (Orosa, 2001), where issues related to the elderly are discussed and taught in courses and workshops. The International Colloquium "El derecho de las personas mayores en el mundo" (The Right of the Elderly in the World) was organized and held in Havana by the International Federation of Associations of Older Persons (FIAPA) and the Center for Research on Aging, Longevity and Health of the Elderly Adult of Cuba. It was cited that older people are the living historical memory of the nation, and that it is very important to understand old age as an authentic stage of human development. In Cuba today there are 276 grandparents' homes and 146 nursing homes dedicated to caring for the elderly, both by providing healthcare and understanding their role in their social environment (Fariñas, 2017).

Engaging the elderly in physical activities

Nowadays in Cuba an increasing number of older people are joining the Physical Culture Therapy Clubs. Thus, it has become necessary for these health clubs to make plans to get senior citizens involved in physical activities. This will keep them away from sedentary habits by engaging them in physical exercises that contribute to keeping their bodies and minds active.

Our elders have a tendency to slow down and spend their old age mainly isolated with their families. However, over the last decade, a growing number of older people are getting involved in physical and recreational activities. This constitutes a significant improvement that can influence their possibilities to attain more space for self-fulfillment. Since 1999, Instituto Nacional de Deporte y Recreación (INDER, the National Institute of Sports, Physical Education and Recreation) Departamento Nacional de Educación Física for adults has laid out methodological orientations for working with older adults. In addition, numerous studies on these important issues are being conducted all over the country, and there are many proposals for programs of activities related to physical culture suitable for people during old age (Ceballos, 2001). The idea is to select activities based on the real possibilities and limitations of the members of these groups as well as their needs, motivations, and social environment. The participants must also be allowed to choose which tasks they prefer to engage in in order to ensure success.

Physical activity is of vital importance for people in this age group because it improves the contractile segments of the body, which are in charge of facilitating coordination, stability, agility, muscular strength, and a defensive response against external stimuli, or simply making a move in a sport or game. And it also aims at reinserting the individual constructively into society where they can interact with other individuals (Diener, Emmons, Larsen, & Griffin 1985). This is a fundamental goal for this stage of life, because it supports the overall quality of life.

Community Grandparents' Circles

The Cuban Ministry of Public Health is also caring for elderly people through the offering of the so-called Grandparents' Circles in coordination with INDER. The Grandparents' Circles or Grandparents' Clubs have become places where seniors meet under the guidance of a family doctor, a nurse, and a physical education instructor. The doctor and the nurse monitor the seniors' vital signs, such as their blood pressure and body temperature, before they start their activities. After the initial clearance, the health professionals determine the intensity of the exercises and activities based on the participants' state of health. Physical, recreational, and cultural activities are offered. Classes for older adults should be conducted in areas where it is feasible to perform them safely for the participants, taking into account the specific characteristics of the people included in each group.

The frequency of involvement in the Grandparent Circle is determined by their conditions and state of health. It ranges from once a week to three times a week or even daily involvement. The execution time will depend on the experience of the group. For instance, for most participants a session may last between 26 and 30 minutes, for the most advanced participants it may last up to 60 minutes. The organizer must include rest breaks to prevent participants from fatigue. The essential contents of the classes should be aimed above all at seeking a greater level of physical and psychological autonomy that enhances sociability toward integration in the community in order to counteract the aging process. Classes should be highly motivational and enjoyable so that participants have fun while exercising. A variety of activities shall be offered to encourage motor memory. When an exercise is introduced, even the most simple, adequate time should be given for each adult to develop their own motor response, since the groups of older adults are diverse and sometimes adaptations to various exercises have to be introduced. Whenever possible, a brief explanation should be made about the benefits reported by the main tasks.

Several studies have been conducted to learn more about the impact that participating in these Grandparents' Circles can have on society. Sánchez and Agüero (1987) and Daure (2015) conducted studies on the level of participation in physical exercises and recreational-cultural activities that were offered to the grandmothers in different circles in Havana. The results found differences in the level of participation in physical exercises and recreational-cultural activities. In this sample 174 older adults from different circles in Havana city were studied and 84.6 percent of participants showed a greater interest in physical exercise than in recreational-cultural activities, especially when participating in class exercise programs. Attention and effort became more constant with the performance of repetitive motions, which led to positive experiences. An improvement in motor skills as well as in the psychological well-being and mental health was reported (Davydov, Stewart, Ritchie, & Chaudieu, 2010; Saavedra & Villalta, 2008).

Daure (2015) obtained similar results in a study that focused on the motivation in 195 elderly members of the Grandparents' Circles of the city of Santa Clara, Cuba. The results obtained were interesting because there was an increase in the interest of practicing physical exercises. These results demonstrate that these activities increase socialization, self-affirmation, self-esteem, reduce the sedentary lifestyle, and raise the overall quality of life. In general, the participating elderly experienced psychological benefits after physical activity practices. They reported an increase in social activities, improvement of self-esteem, reduction of their sedentary lifestyle, and a rise in their overall quality of life.

It was found that positive psychological and social improvements correlated in those older adults attending classes for a prolonged period of time, and when they were more active for more hours a day outside of their homes. They also kept in touch with friends, acquaintances, and relatives more often. In addition, these elderly had developed greater control of their bodies and a certain degree of re-socialization, when compared with those who registered in the Grandparents' Circles for the first time (Cañizares, 2009).

It is important to emphasize that interest in recreational and cultural activities was maintained by all older adults studied (Lahera, 2015). They attended parties, picnics, excursions, movies; visited exhibitions, museums, theaters, craft shows, and more. This gave them further opportunities to interact with people of their age and form interpersonal relationships. In general, these adults experience psychological benefits after being involved in physical activity practices, including increased socialization, improvement of self-esteem, reduction of sedentary lifestyle, and a greater quality of life. Socio-cultural activities in these Grandparents' Circles are aimed at combatting isolation and loneliness, increasing self-confidence, personal satisfaction, and self-esteem. Occupying once free time with cultural and recreational programs eliminates barriers and provides a range of freely chosen action by these adults (Woodman, Akehurst, Hardy, & Beattie, 2010; Diener, Emmons, Larsen & Griffin, 1985).

When planning the various activities for older adults in these Grand-parents' Circles, it is important to adapt to the group's abilities, the conditions of the place, and the choice of educational/didactic treatments that allow all participants to participate at their individual levels. The activities carried out are comprised of two groups: *basic activities* and *complementary activities*. Basic activities include gymnastics with and without implements, soft gymnastics, games, body expression, aerobic activities (low impact gymnastics, jogging, hiking, etc.), rhythmic activities, exercises with small weights, and relaxation with self-massage. The complementary activities include walking, aquatic activities (gymnastics and water games, swimming, bathing in the sea), traditional dances, popular games and adapted sports, recreational festivals, gymnastic compositions, sports-cultural encounters, and social gatherings. The objective is to have fun while getting fit and combatting the slowing down of the aging process.

The aging retired athlete

In Cuba today there is also a great concern about supporting former athletes in their aging processes. The Cuban government has expressed concern about the quality of life and the psychological well-being of retired athletes. Thus, all centers of sports and sport medicine in the country are offering psychological consultations as part of the treatment for healthy aging and combatting the suffering that often goes hand in hand with the *de-training* process. Generally, these centers include consultations in the areas of dermatology, cardiology, psychology, orthopedics, physio-therapy, dentistry, osteopathy, among others. Athletes who attend the clinics have their medical history analyzed and benefit from the services provided for them.

In these sport medicine centers the older population has access not only to healthcare but can also participate in physical activities, ranging from gymnastics, popular games and sports, rhythmic activities, relaxation techniques, outdoor work, contact with nature or with the aquatic environment. In the case of retired athletes, the care is more specialized and performed in conjunction with their specific de-training plan.

At the moment, research is conducted to analyze which psycho-educational guidelines are best offered to address the psychological symptoms of retired athletes during menopause in the phase of de-training. The results show that former athletes are benefitting from this specific assistance (Gómez, 2016). Gómez, Delisle, and Cañizares (2016) emphasize that menopause is a natural stage in the life of a woman, which can be accompanied by uncomfortable symptoms, due to the reduction of estrogen levels, and thus can affect the overall well-being of some women. Women retired from sports, in particular, may face further physical and psychological disorders.

At this stage in the aging process, athletes may face many crises, including changes in life, new interests, new relationships, friendships, menopause, and other general health conditions related to the aging process. Thus, it is of great value that the process of de-training is addressed in a special way for the former athletes. One of the issues that could cause physical and psychological discomfort is menopause for females. Specific support and psychological care, from diagnosis to intervention, could support the well-being of women and high-performance retired athletes. When the doctor and psychologist analyze the sports records of these former athletes, they have an idea about the main characteristics of the personality of the subject, their sports results, goals, family life, as well as their socio-economic status and their personal medical history. These sport records, which are kept for every athlete in the country, are great guiding tools to make adequate diagnoses, and they can greatly assist in the development of adequate psychological intervention programs.

Research sample, methodology, and findings on the retired athletes' involvement in physical activities and psychological programs

The psychological attention provided to retired athletes requires the analysis of the different environmental and subjective responses that affect their lives. These athletes need guidance, support, and treatment; and physicians and psychologists play an important role. They can enhance the psycho-emotional support by promoting an environment of security, acceptance, and respect. Special instruments were created to evaluate and organize intervention programs with the objective of increasing the psychological well-being as these retired athletes are facing the next stage in their lives, away from active sports. The medical and psychological care in this process focuses mainly on issues related to self-adjustment, evaluation of anxiety levels, depression, motivation, aspiration levels, and the overall psychological well-being of the former athletes.

In this study, we analyzed a group of high-performing female basketball athletes (n=23) from the national team, who were diagnosed by the Institute of Sports Medicine to be in the menopausal stage. Their average age was about 54 years of age (Gómez, 2016), and they had often received psychological treatment to address alterations in their mood, dreams, and sex life.

The objective of the research was to apply a system of educational actions to support the psychological symptoms faced during menopause.

In addition, a psychologist on site provided important information on the characteristics of the personality of these ex-athletes during their active participation on the National Basketball Team. The following educational activities were selected to support the psychological care of high-performance female athletes in order to promote greater well-being and a better quality of life:

- *Preventive measures*: Taking into consideration that menopause can lead to personal, social, and relationship crises which effect women differently, specialized information and professional care has been designed to help.
- *Developmental measures*: These actions are designed to promote new transformations and a clear understanding by the ex-athletes of what they are going though, so that they can actively, critically, and creatively change their own attitudes and behavior.
- *Differentiated measures*: Special attention is paid to diversity and the individualistic characteristics of each person.
- *Flexibility*: Actions prescribed to the ex-athletes need to be adjusted to their individual personality traits.

In order to apply the above stated measures, the methodology for the development of psycho-educational care for ex-athletic women during menopausal stage (developed by Gómez, 2016) was used. They include:

- the development of empathy by fostering an environment of trust and security between psychologist and the patient, here the ex-athletes;
- the improvement of the level of knowledge on the part of the participants;
- the disclosure of the importance of proper performance of sports de-training during the work sessions;
- the establishment of appropriate mechanisms to achieve active participation of all involved in this process;
- the use of cognitive-behavioral therapy techniques with the aim of being able to restructure ideas/ beliefs and to modify erroneous attitudes, as well as to recover a sense of personal value and improvement of self-perception, providing clear direction and meaning for life during menopausal stage;
- the use of coping mechanisms to reduce the symptoms brought on by menopause in the short, medium and long term applying various psycho-physiological techniques such as relaxation and breathing;
- taking into account the personal and professional goals of the individuals, and thus favoring the development of the subjective well-being;
- working with the ex-athletes in small groups, which contributes to their personal-social growth.

These described techniques were used to achieve the overall objectives of the study including the use of group dynamics, video conferences (entitled *Learning about Phytoestrogens*), as well as participation in the workshop *My Life: My Sex Life in Menopause*. Applying these above outlined techniques it was possible to offer retired athletes information about the physiological and psychological alterations caused by menopause. Tools are used to improve the mood alterations and the depression related to the climacteric stage. And social skills were developed to mitigate the psychological symptoms related to menopause, such as improving self-esteem, mood, depression, and refuting beliefs and misinformation regarding the climacteric process.

The outcome of this study reports that 100 percent of the interviewees showed satisfaction with the support they received. Their willingness to follow these individually designed actions will support them during the menopausal and declining stages in their lives, including their de-training. Gómez (2016), La Voi (2011), and Brea and Acosta (2000) also have obtained similar results in their research studies that stress the role of women's social rights. Hence, the research cited in this chapter, where physical and psychological measures were used to help individuals in their aging process, is of great significance. The results confirm an increase in the overall health and well-being of the elderly has been achieved for the population at large as well as the ex-athletes in their de-training stages.

Conclusions

Research has shown that the regular practice of physical activity offers benefits for physical and mental health. A remarkable stimulation of motor skills and abilities has been observed, as well as a reduction in sedentary habits. In addition, cognitive activity has also improved through the involvement in table games and bowling, for example. Mental skills are stimulated when playing games or engaging in exercises, for example, through analysis and memorization of numbers, colors, names, among others. Self-esteem is improved as well, and the adults experience reaffirmation as being an active agent in their environment.

The Cuban government provides care for its elderly and has gained great experience with the creation of Grandparents' Circles in the community. Grandparents' Circles are spaces where older people gather in groups, accompanied by their family doctor, a nurse, and a professor of Physical Culture. Physical and psychological benefits are assessed following the physical activity practiced. Results show that engaging in these activities improves overall health, increases socialization and self-esteem, reduces physical inactivity, and increases the overall quality of life.

In addition, since the Cuban government has expressed concern about the quality of life and especially the psychological well-being of aging retired athletes, these individuals have received special treatment at the centers of sports medicine. These special consultations aim to assist with a smooth and healthy de-training process, including support during the menopausal stage of former top-level female athletes. Specific psycho-educational activities have been developed to assist in this important phase in the aging process, including self-help activities and participation in group workshops. Overall, engaging in regular physical activities has been proven to be extremely beneficial during the overall aging process.

References

Beutel, M. E., Glaesmer, H., Decker, O., Fischbeck, S., & Brahler, E. (2009). Life satisfaction, distress, and resiliency across the life span of women. *The Journal of North American Menopause Society, 16*(12), 1132–1138.

Brea, C. T. & Acosta, R. V. (2000) *Social Rights of Woman III Pan-American Congress for women. "Memories."* Ministry of Education, Culture and Sports. Venezuela. (National Institute of Sports, Physical Education and Recreation).

Cañizares, M. (2009). *Psychology in physical activity. Its application in physical education, sport, recreation and rehabilitation.* Havana, Editorial Sports.

Ceballos, J. (2001). *The elderly and physical activity.* Ebook. UCCFD Manuel Fajardo, pp. 23–34.

Daure, J. (2015). La actividad física en la tercera edad. In Gavotto, H., Cañizares, M., & Gavotto, O. (2015). *Intervención psicológica en el deporte, la actividad física y recreación.* Mexico: Editorial PEARSON, pp. 91–92.

Davydov, D. M., Stewart, R., Ritchie, K., & Chaudieu, I. (2010). Resilience and mental health. *Clinical Psychology Review, 30*(5), 479–495.

Diener, E., Emmons, R., Larsen, R., & Griffin, S. (1985). The satisfaction with life scale. *Journal of Personality Assessment, 49*(1), 71–75.

Fariñas, L. (2017, 4 April). Hablan las voces mayores. *Periódico Granma,* p. 2.

Gavotto, H., Cañizares, M., & Gavotto, O. (2015). *Intervención psicológica en el deporte, la actividad física y recreación.* Mexico. Editorial PEARSON.

Gómez, Z. (2016). Propuesta de acciones psicoeducaivas para el control de los síntomas del climaterio en atletas retiradas. La Habana. 150 h. Tesis no publicada (en opción al grado académico de máster en Psicología del deporte). UCCFD "Manuel Fajardo," La Habana, Cuba.

Gómez, Z., Delisle, M., & Cañizares, M. (2016). Acciones psicoeducaivas para el control de los síntomas del climaterioen atletas retiradas. Report in the Primer Simposio de Cultura Física Terapéutica, diciembre, UCCFD "Manuel Fajardo," La Habana, Cuba.

Henry, T. (1990). *Higher stages of human development perspectives on adult growth.* Edited by C. Alexander & E. Jlanger. New York: Oxford University.

Lahera, A. (2015). Modification of personal motivational configurations of older adults through the practice of physical exercises of the ex – convent "San Agustín," Habana Vieja. *Acción, 7*(13), 3–6.

La Voi, N. M. (2011). Trends in gender-related research in sport and exercise psychology. *Revista Iberoamericana de Psicología del Ejercicio y el deporte, 6*(4).

Orosa, F. T. (2001). *La tercera edad y la familia. Una mirada desde el envejecimiento.* La Habana : Editorial Felix Varela.

Saavedra, E. & Villalta, M. (2008). Medición de las características resilientes, un estudio comparativo en personas entre 15 y 65 años. *Liberabit, 14,* 31–40.

Sánchez Acosta, M. E. & Agüero, E. (1987) Análisis del nivel de participación en ejercicios físicas y actividades culturales en los círculos de abuelos del municipio Plaza de la Revolución. Informe de investigación, UCCFD "Manuel Fajardo," La Habana, Cuba.

Tolstij, A. (1989). *El hombre y la edad.* Moscú: Editorial Progreso.

Woodman, T., Akehurst, S., Hardy, L., & Beattie, S. (2010). Self-confidence and performance: a little self-doubt helps. *Psychology of Sport and Exercise, 11*(6), 467–470.

Chapter 8

Aging and fitness programs
Influencing factors, professional intervention, and challenges in Spain

María Dolores González-Rivera

Demographic indicators, longevity, and health in Spain

The number of people aged 65 and over reached the figure of 8.6 million, and represents 18.5 percent of Spain's total population. Life expectancy at birth is 82.87 years (85.58 years for women and 80.08 years for men) (Spanish National Institute of Statistics, 2016). Spain is one of the European Union countries with the highest number of older adults and highest levels of life expectancy at age 65 (Abellán & Pujol, 2015).

The White Paper on active aging, edited by the Ministry of Health, Social Policy and Equality in Spain (Causapié, Balbontín, Porras, & Mateo, 2011) highlights various trends for consideration when examining the needs and formulating proposals regarding these demographic challenges and their consequences. In addition to declining fertility and increasing life expectancy, these emerging trends include a regional imbalance in the distribution of older adults. The regions of Castilla y León, Galicia, Asturias, Aragón, and the Basque Country are the regions with the oldest populations, where older adults account for over 20 percent of the population. The Canary Islands, Balearic Islands, and Murcia are the regions with the lowest rates, with under 15 percent. Andalucia, Catalonia, and Madrid are the regions with the most older adults concentrated in urban areas (Abellán & Pujol, 2015).

In addition, Spain experienced a spectacular increase in emigration in the late twentieth century, including migration by older people seeking climate comfort, especially in the last decade. This has led to a significant increase in the number of European retirees in Spain's Mediterranean coastal areas and islands. This trend is also due to the low cost of living and the availability of health and leisure facilities (Causapié, Balbontín, Porras, & Mateo, 2011). Furthermore, the *Federation of Pensioners and Retired People* report of Comisiones Obreras (2016) highlights increasing emigration for work among the Spanish population since the beginning of the economic crisis, and the departure of the country's young Spanish and foreign population.

Another important factor in the process of aging is the changing patterns of illness and death in the twentieth century, with chronic diseases affecting more than 19 million people in Spain and with a prevalence that is particularly concentrated in people 55+ and increases with age (EsCrónicos, 2016). According to the *Spanish national health survey 2011/12* (Ministry of Health, Social Services and Equality, n.d.), the most common chronic problems and illnesses among people aged 65 and over are: Arthritis and rheumatism (52.9 percent), high blood pressure (47.1 percent), chronic lumbar back pain (32.5 percent), high cholesterol (32.2 percent), chronic cervical back pain (29.2 percent), varicose veins in the legs (23.8 percent), and diabetes (19.3 percent). This survey also reveals a high percentage of people with a sedentary lifestyle (42.2 percent of those between 65 and 74 years old; 56.2 percent of those between 75 and 84 years old, and over 76.9 percent of those aged 85+). Approximately 44 percent of adults believe that their state of health is good or very good, with this belief being more prevalent among men than women.

Sports habits, barriers, and the needs of older adults

Sports habits, demands and barriers to older people engaging in sport and physical activity (SPA) are factors influencing the adequate design and improvement of services and programs adapted to this population group. Therefore, an evaluation of the program offerings will provide insights in the identification of future needs and implications (Martín, Martínez, & Ferro, 2012).

Surveys conducted by the Spanish government on the sport and physical activity habits of the Spanish population found a progressive increase in SPA among people aged 65+, from 8 percent in 2000 (García-Ferrando, 2001) to 30 percent obtained in 2015 (National Sports Council (NSC), 2015). However, involvement in SPA remains insufficient (Salinas, Cocca, Mohamed, & Viciana, 2010) with older adults having lower percentages compared to other demographic groups and different sports habits (González-Rivera, Martín, Jiménez-Beatty, Campos-Izquierdo, & del Hierro, 2010).

The most recent survey of Spaniards' activity habits (NSC, 2015) found that the most popular types of sports among adults aged 65+ are low impact gymnastics, swimming, hiking, and mountaineering, with football and basketball being the least popular. A larger proportion of older adults engage in SPA on working days rather than on weekends and holidays. In addition, the study by Jiménez-Beatty et al. (2009) indicates that 36 percent of older people engage in physical activity in a sports facility, 39 percent in activity centers (such as homes for senior citizens), 14 percent in their home, 4.4 percent in parks, and 6.9 percent do so in other natural areas.

The main reasons why older people engage in physical activity are to keep fit, improve health, enjoy leisure, or for entertainment and relaxation. However, the main reasons why they are not more physically active are increasing age, state of health, lack of interest, and lack of time (NSC, 2015), meaning that the greatest barrier is the state of health due to the aging process (Moscoso et al., 2009). Other barriers include the characteristics and social environments of older adults, the shortcomings of facilities with varying differences in certain Spanish regions, shortcomings in the range of activities available, and the level of income and education (Jiménez-Beatty et al., 2009; Moscoso et al., 2009; Martínez et al., 2010; Martín et al., 2012).

González-Rivera, Martín, and Jiménez-Beatty (2009) find that physical exercise services offered in a gymnasium and swimming pool are subject to the highest demand from older adults, followed by outdoor sports and physical activities in urban areas. Another reason for increased SPA among older adults is a recommendation from a doctor, since various studies have concluded that active older people have received medical advice to do SPA more frequently than those who are less active. This advice is also more prevalent among older adults who already engage in SPA or those who would like to, than among older adults who neither do SPA nor wish to (Martínez, Jiménez-Beatty, Santacruz, Martín, & Rivero, 2011; Martín et al., 2012).

Another important aspect of older adults' needs in terms of promoting, organizing, and engaging in adequate SPA programs is the presence of SPA professionals, as this can be an influential factor in reducing barriers to engaging in SPA (Campos-Izquierdo, Jiménez-Beatty, González-Rivera, Martín, & del Hierro, 2011). Various studies have shown that the vast majority of older adults want professionals when doing these activities (Fernández et al., 2008). This need, however, may sometimes constitute a barrier itself, since researchers in Spain have also found that the majority of these professionals do not have appropriate SPA qualifications. As a result, the quality and professionalism of services are not guaranteed in these cases, and could pose a challenge to the individuals' safety, health and other social and educational benefits (Campos-Izquierdo, González-Rivera, & Taks, 2016).

Professional intervention in SPA and health education

Investigators in Spain and in other countries have found that among older adults, having previously done sports increases the chances of doing so later in life, and that this intervention is decisive at advanced stages of life (Moscoso et al., 2009). Adequate training in physical education and in extracurricular physical-sports activities is therefore a crucial factor.

Furthermore, an increase in the number of hours of physical education taught in school per week (there are fewer hours in Spain than in other European countries) and an adequate and effective link to extracurricular physical-sports activities is a necessary foundation in order to achieve healthy lifelong habits (González-Rivera and Campos-Izquierdo, 2014).

In Spain, many older adults are, unfortunately, ill-informed about the types and amount of SPA that are most beneficial to them. It is, therefore, essential to provide information and advice on healthy lifestyle alternatives to enable them to change their behavior and to maximize the likelihood of successful active aging (Romo-Pérez, Schwingel, & Chodzko-Zajko, 2011). Thus, personalized and efficient professional intervention of SPA professionals is of utmost importance, based on the individual characteristics, needs, abilities and the type of possible illnesses of the participants (Campos-Izquierdo, Jiménez-Beatty, González-Rivera, Martín, & del Hierro, 2011). Accordingly, if SPA is not supervised and developed by a SPA professional, the benefits for the elderly population will not be achieved and might have counter-productive effects on their health (González-Rivera, Campos-Izquierdo, & Martínez, 2012a).

Studies in Spain have shown that many SPA services offered do not have professionals with appropriate SPA qualifications (Campos-Izquierdo, 2010; 2016). The National Sports Council (NSC, 2009) also says that there is a lack of professional recognition for professionals responsible for implementing SPA programs for older adults. Likewise, a research project, financed by Ministry of Science and Innovation in Spain (DEP2009-12828) and led by Campos-Izquierdo (2013) on employment, found that 41 percent of people working with SPA programs with older adults do not have any SPA qualifications. This was compared to 59 percent who do (González-Rivera, Campos-Izquierdo, & Martínez, 2012a). The majority of these workers (72.9 percent) undertook one or several lifelong learning activities in the past four years, with the most common being courses (65.7 percent) (González-Rivera, Campos-Izquierdo, & Martínez, 2012b). Furthermore, Campos-Izquierdo (2013) found that 77.8 percent of these people have a contract with an institution and 10.8 percent are self-employed or entrepreneurs, although 11.3 percent had no contract. It was also found that 62 percent have a permanent contract and 38 percent have a temporary contract (Campos-Izquierdo, 2013). In the private institutions where these people work, 42.1 percent have no SPA qualification, and 30.6 percent did not have a SPA qualification in public institutions (González-Rivera, Campos-Izquierdo, & Martínez, 2012a).

Given this context of inadequate training and employment status of SPA professionals, regional governments in Spain have recently enacted laws to regulate sport professions to ensure the safety and health of those engaging in SPA. The most recent regional law (*Law 6/2016 of November 24*) regulates sport professions in the region of Madrid. According to this Law, a physical trainer is a professional, who among other tasks, engages in the rehabilitation, retraining and/or re-education of people with injuries and pathologies (diagnosed and/or prescribed by a doctor) by means of physical-sports activities and exercises adapted to their characteristics and needs, and the preparation, advice, planning, development and technical-scientific evaluation of physical-sports activities and physical exercises aimed at improving the quality of life and health of older adults.

This Law further stipulates that a physical trainer also performs activities and tasks involved in sports initiation and instruction, guidance, sports entertainment and basic physical group exercises with older adults, and that a physical trainer must possess a degree in Physical Activity and Sport Sciences. This enactment of law and policy is a step in the right direction.

Differences in accessing SPA resources—gender and social status

Age, socio-economic status, and gender are factors that discriminate in sports (Jiménez-Beatty, González-Rivera, Martín, del Hierro & Martínez, 2008). Researchers at the Institute for Women (2006) found that there was an absence of physical exercise and sport activities to a greater extent among older women (who engaged solely in housework), retired women, and those with a low educational level and with a low income level. In addition, Martínez et al. (2010) found that higher social status increased the probability of SPA being present in older adults' lifestyles.

Likewise, Martín, González-Rivera, Campos-Izquierdo, Del Hierro, and Jiménez-Beatty (2010) found different profiles for the SPA habits of older people according to their social status. People of high social standing do SPA mainly in companies and associations, which they mostly walk to, and carry out physical exercise programs or other physical activities (30 percent), for an average of 3 hours a week. People of medium social standing do SPA mainly in centers for older adults and municipal sports facilities (which they mostly walk to) and engage in physical exercise programs or other physical activities (40 percent), for an average of 3 hours a week. Almost all older adults with a lower social standing do SPA in centers for older adults (which is usually free of charge) and municipal sports centers, which they almost all walk to, for 2 or 3 hours a week.

Gender also shapes activity patterns. According to the Institute for Women (2006), the decline in frequency of sport engagement increases with age and is more noticeable among males. Activity levels also decrease for women but there is some increase in later life when they are freed of childcare and have additional leisure time. Martín, González-Rivera, Campos-Izquierdo, Del Hierro, and Jiménez-Beatty (2010) and Martínez et al. (2009) found that unlike other age groups, women over 65 have higher percentages of engaging in SPA than their male counterparts. According to the Institute for Women (2006), women are increasingly involved with SPA, and they create their own types of sport and physical activity that they enjoy. To gain further insights, an analysis of the differences and similarities in the gendered sports culture is essential for a successful policy and provision of SPA to ensure greater participation for all in the older population (Martín, González-Rivera, Campos-Izquierdo, & Hierro and Jiménez-Beatty, 2010).

The studies by Martín, Moscoso, and Pedrajas (2013) and Martín, González-Rivera, Campos-Izquierdo, Del Hierro, and Jiménez-Beatty (2010) found that motivations related to health and enjoyment of sport are most frequently mentioned by both sexes, and women value motivations related to entertainment and social relationships to a greater extent. Interestingly, men respond that their motivation is habit or that they have always done sports more frequently than women. Furthermore, the studies by Martín et al. (2010, 2012) find that older people who do not engage but are interested in SPA mainly ask for programs involving physical exercise and water activities. Although women, to a lesser extent, prefer activities involving oriental gymnastics and activities with music, men prefer competitive activities or self-organized outdoor activities.

SPA programs for seniors in Spain

Some progress has been made toward the implementation of SPA programs by the various Spanish government bodies and institutions (Pont & Soler, 2011). In order to promote universal access to quality sports for the population, the NSC (2010) launched the *Comprehensive plan for physical activity and sport*, in close collaboration with autonomous regional governments, local authorities, universities, and other ministerial organizations, as well as with the private sector. This plan covers the period 2010 to 2020, and one of its priority objectives is systematic engagement in physical exercise among older adults through the implementation of programs that meet their needs. This includes healthy pro-aging policies in various areas—such as health, sports, tourism, urbanism, and more—which facilitates the establishment of multidisciplinary teams, led by a specialist in physical education. The *Comprehensive plan for physical activity and sport for older adults* has been formulated (NSC, 2009) which contains various types of programs that have been successfully implemented in different regions of Spain. These include:

- *socio-motor programs*, which aim to use SPA to maintain and improve the participants' general physical condition, their cognitive abilities and social relationships;

- *fitness programs* aimed at autonomous older adults with a good degree of mobility, which place more emphasis on improving their physical condition;
- *outdoors programs for seniors* using the footpaths in the various regions of Spain and the country's geography and climate;
- *programs for frail senior adults for the prevention of dependence*, where an interdisciplinary team performs the initial intervention. This involves a final check by a medical team and a SPA professional, with a degree in Physical Activity and Sports Sciences, who is responsible for carrying out the program.

Also noteworthy are the programs provided by the Institute for Older People and Social Services (affiliated with the Ministry of Health, Social Services and Equality), which has expanded its range in recent years to include physical activities. Finally, there are sports programs, in which sports clubs and their respective federations organize and promote sport for seniors, adapting rules and creating categories according to age (Pont & Soler, 2011). Furthermore, the Ministry of Health and Consumer Affairs (2005) produced the *Strategy for nutrition, physical activity and prevention of obesity* (the NAOS Strategy), aimed at improving dietary habits and promoting regular SPA among all citizens. The Ministry of Health, Social Services and Equality (2014) also implemented the *Strategy for health promotion and prevention in the national health system* (within the framework of chronicity in the Spanish health services), and among its objectives is the promotion of active and healthy aging among older adults through a comprehensive intervention focusing on healthy lifestyles. And it is noteworthy that autonomous regional Spanish governments are now implementing healthy programs, such as: the *Comprehensive plan for the promotion of health through physical activity and healthy eating* in Catalonia (Government of Catalonia, 2008); the *Comprehensive plan for the promotion of sports and physical activity* in Extremadura (Government of Extremadura, 2009); the *Healthy Galicia plan for promoting physical activity* in Galicia (Government of Galicia, 2011); the *Active aging strategy of the Valencian community* (Government of the Valencian Community, 2013) and the *Enforma program* of the Madrid Region (Government of Madrid Community, 2017).

Future plans and needs—strategies, implications, and challenges

The Spanish government is aware of the limitations of promoting SPA among the older population and is proposing four strategic initiatives to be carried out in the short, medium, and long term as part of the *Comprehensive plan for the promotion of sport and physical activity among older adults* (NSC, 2009). These strategic initiatives, which are set out below, are in line with the various implications and specific challenges identified in research, as well as by other Spanish institutional bodies.

One strategic area is the promotion of healthy habits among older adults. Because the research has found that these people would probably be regular practitioners if SPA services were properly organized (González-Rivera, Martín, and Jiménez-Beatty, 2009; Martín et al., 2012), it is important to take into account the various circumstances, expectations, needs and motivations of the elderly (Pont & Soler, 2011). Hence, a diversified and adapted range of programs according to the individual motivations, degree of dependence, social status, and gender should be offered (Dapia, 2012; NSC, 2009).There is also a need for initiatives that raise awareness of the existence of facilities available, i.e., through the media, in health centers and centers where older adults meet, and more (Ministry of Health and Consumer Affairs, 2005; NSC, 2009).

Another strategic area is training for professionals who work on SPA programs for older adults. Because researchers in Spain have found that older adults want activities to be directed by SPA professionals, a range of SPA services must be created that meet this demand. Such initiative will improve the quality of programs offered and also prevent possible errors or accidents, because of absence of SPA professionals or the individual's lack of training or ability to perform this task (Fernández et al., 2008). An adequate professional intervention and performance depend on these professionals having the appropriate SPA training and qualification that ensure good practices, health, education and safety of all citizens engaging in SPA (Campos-Izquierdo, 2016). Therefore, it is necessary to include competence and content about SPA for older adults into the curricula of degree programs in Physical Activity and Sports Sciences (Campos-Izquierdo & Martín-Acero, 2016).

Another strategic area is the adaptation of natural and urban spaces that encourage sports, by promoting healthy cities with multidisciplinary teams, including municipal officials, town planners, managers of leisure and sport activities, educators, and more, at an autonomous regional and municipal level (Ministry of Health and Consumer Affairs, 2005; NSC, 2009). Furthermore, architectural barriers that hinder accessibility need to be eliminated in order to ensure the safety of older adults in the sports centers concerned (NSC, 2009). In addition, a study by Dapia (2012) highlights the urgent need for improved SPA services for older adults in rural areas, by providing an efficient intra-municipal transportation system or alternatively, by decentralizing community leisure programs and providing activities in all municipalities.

Another strategic area is the inclusion of healthy pro-aging policies with the participation of various sectors, including health, sports, urbanism, and tourism at different levels. Government, autonomous regional governments, local institutions, universities, research groups, and more need to establish an overall framework for action. The creation of multi-disciplinary teams should include physical trainers, doctors, educators, geriatricians, social workers, nurses, physiotherapists, occupational therapists, sociologists, economists, and others, who can guarantee the optimal implementation, development and follow-up of designed initiatives (NSC, 2009). Coordinated initiatives by sports organizations with health centers and medical personnel should be promoted along with a simultaneous focus on improving public health in the various regions of Spain (Martín et al., 2012; Martínez, Jiménez-Beatty, Santacruz, Martín, & Rivero, 2011). This is stipulated in the law that was devised for the Madrid Autonomous Region (*Law 6/2016 of 24 November*) which regulates the exercise of sports professions whereby SPA programs for older adults must be coordinated effectively with primary healthcare physicians and physical activity specialists. Designing exercise programs fit for the elderly, educating SPA specialists, spreading policy, and creating laws as described above, will greatly support the growing older population in Spain in experiencing a quality aging process.

References

Abellán, A. & Pujol, R. (2015). *Un perfil de las personas mayores en España, 2015. Indicadores estadísticos básicos.* Madrid: Informes Envejecimiento en red no. 10. Retrieved from http://envejecimiento.csic.es/documentos/documentos/enred-indicadoresbasicos15.pdf.

Campos-Izquierdo, A. (2010). *Dirección de recursos humanos en las organizaciones de la actividad física y del deporte.* Madrid: Síntesis.

Campos-Izquierdo, A. (Coord.). (2013). *Research project: Occupational and organisational structure of human resources of physical activity and sports in Spain.* Madrid: Spanish Ministry of Science and Innovation.

Campos-Izquierdo, A. (2016). La formación de los profesionales de actividad física y deporte en España. *Movimento, 22* (4), 1351–1364.

Campos-Izquierdo, A. & Marín-Acero, R. (2016). Percepción de las competencias profesionales de los graduados en Ciencias de la Actividad Física y del Deporte. *Revista de Psicología del Deporte, 25* (2), 339–346.

Campos-Izquierdo, A., González-Rivera, M.D., & Taks, M. (2016). Multifunctionality and occupations of sport and physical activity professionals in Spain. *European Sport Management Quarterly, 16* (1), 106–126.

Campos-Izquierdo, A., Jiménez-Beatty, J.E., González-Rivera, M.D., Martín, M. & del Hierro, D. (2011). Demanda y percepción del monitor de la personas mayores en la actividad física y deporte en España. *Revista de Psicología del Deporte, 20* (1), 61–77.

Causapié, P., Balbontín, A., Porras, M., & Mateo, A. (Coords.). (2011). *Envejecimiento activo. Libro Blanco.* Madrid: Ministry of Health, Social Policy and Equality.

Dapia, M. (2012). Leisure patterns and needs of the elderly in rural Galicia (Spain). *Educational Gerontology, 38*(2), 138–145.

EsCrónicos (2016). *III barómetro Escrónicos. Encuesta sobre la calidad de la asistencia sanitaria a los pacientes crónicos en España.* Retrieved from www.escronicos.com/images/barometro/presentacion-2016.pdf.

Federation of Pensioners and Retired People of Comisiones Obreras (2016). *Observatorio social de personas mayores. Para un envejecimiento activo.* Madrid: Comisiones Obreras. Retrieved from www.1mayo.ccoo.es/nova/files/1018/ObservatorioSocial2016.pdf.

Fernández, I., Campos-Izquierdo, A., Jiménez-Beatty, J.E., González-Rivera, M.D., Martín, M., & del Hierro (2008). La demanda de los recursos humanos por parte de las personas mayores que practican actividad física en España. *Cultura, Ciencia y Deporte, Suppl. 3*, 16.

García-Ferrando, M. (2001). *Los españoles y el deporte: Prácticas y comportamientos en la última década del siglo XX.* Madrid: NSC.

González-Rivera, M.D. & Campos-Izquierdo, A. (2014). *Intervención docente en educación física en secundaria y en el deporte escolar.* Madrid: Síntesis.

González-Rivera, M.D., Campos-Izquierdo, A., & Martínez, G. (2012a). The training of the monitors that work in physical activity and spot programmes with older adults in Spain. *Journal of Aging and Physical Activity, Suppl. 20*, 92–93.

González-Rivera, M.D., Campos-Izquierdo, A., & Martínez, G. (2012b). Formación permanente de los monitores de actividad física y deporte con personas mayores en España. In R. Escobar and A. Sánchez (Dir.), *VII Congreso Internacional de Ciencias del Deporte* (p. 229). Granada: Asociación Española de Ciencias del Deporte.

González-Rivera, M.D., Martín, M., & Jiménez-Beatty, J.E. (2009). Estudios de las demandas de servicios de actividad física de las personas mayores en España. Características organizativas. In A. Vilanova, J. Castillo, A. Fraile, M. González, J. Martínez, N. Puig ... S. Soler (Comps.), *Deporte, Salud y Medioambiente* (pp. 449–464). Madrid: Esteban Sanz.

González-Rivera, M.D., Martín, M., Jiménez-Beatty, J.E., Campos-Izquierdo, A., & del Hierro, D. (2010). *Los hábitos de actividad física de las personas mayores en España y condición social. Apunts. Educación Física y Deporte, 101*, 83–84.

Government of Catalonia (2008). *Comprehensive plan for the promotion of health through physical activity and healthy eating.* Barcelona: Government of Catalonia. Retrieved from http://salutweb.gencat.cat/web/.content/home/ambits_tematics/linies_dactuacio/salut_i_qualitat/salut_publica/paas/documents/arxius/paas.pdf.

Government of Extremadura (2009). *Comprehensive plan for the promotion of sports and physical activity.* Mérida: Junta de Extremadura. Retrieved from http://deportextremadura.gobex.es/images/Documentos/Plan%20Integral%20Deporte.pdf.

Government of Galicia (2011). *Healthy Galicia plan for promoting physical activity.* Retrieved from http://galiciasaudable.xunta.gal/c/document_library/get_file?folderId=1852845&name=DLFE-11464.pdf.

Government of Madrid Community (2017). *Enforma programme.* Retrieved from www.madrid.org/sumadeporte/index.php/actividades-instalaciones/programmea-enforma.

Government of the Valencian Community (2013). *Active aging strategy of the Valencian Community.* Valencia: Government of the Valencian Community.

Retrieved from http://cuidatecv.es/wp-content/uploads/2014/01/ESTRATEGIA-ENVEJECIMIENTO-ACTIVO-EN-LA-CV-2013-CAST-11.pdf.

Institute for Women (2006). *Actitudes y prácticas deportivas de las mujeres en España (1990–2005)*. Madrid: Institute for Women. Retrieved from www. inmujer.gob.es/areasTematicas/estudios/serieEstudios/docs/92practdeportivas. pdf.

Jiménez-Beatty, J.E., González-Rivera, M.D., Martín, M., del Hierro, D., & Martínez, J. (2008). Hábitos de actividad física y demandas de servicios de actividad física de las mujeres adultas. *efdeportes, Revista Digital, 118*. Retrieved from www.efdeportes.com/efd118/habitos-de-actividad-fisica-mujeres-adultas.htm.

Jiménez-Beatty, J.E., Martínez, J., Campos-Izquierdo, A., del Hierro, D., Martín, M., & González-Rivera, M.D. (2009). Los centros y espacios de actividad física utilizados por las personas mayores en España. In A. Vilanova, J. Castillo, A. Fraile, M. González, J. Martínez, N. Puig ... S. Soler (Comps.), *Deporte, Salud y Medioambiente* (pp. 457–455). Madrid: Esteban Sanz.

Martín, M., González-Rivera, M.D., Campos-Izquierdo, A., Del Hierro, D., & Jiménez-Beatty, J.E. (2010). Expectativas de la demanda latente de actividad física de las mujeres y hombres mayores en España. *Cultura, Ciencia y Deporte, 15* (5), 141– 150.

Martín, M., Martínez, J., & Ferro, S. (2012). Impulsando la práctica de actividades físico-deportivas en la vejez. *Anduli, 11*, 23–39.

Martín, M., Martínez, J., Serrano, J.A., Jiménez-Beatty, J.E., Santacruz, J.A., & Rivero, A. (2012). Associations among physician advice, physical activity, and socio-demographic groups in older Spanish adults. *Canadian Journal on Aging, 31* (3) 349–356.

Martín, M., Moscoso, D., & Pedrajas, N. (2013). Gender differences in motivations to practice physical activity and sport in old age. *Revista Internacional de Medicina y Ciencias de la Actividad Física y el Deporte, 13* (49), 121–129.

Martínez, J., Jiménez-Beatty, J.E., Campos, A., Del Hierro, D., Martín, M., & González-Rivera, M.D. (2010). Barreras organizativas y sociales para la práctica de la actividad física en la vejez. *Motricidad. European Journal of Human Movement, 19*, 13–35.

Martínez, J., Jiménez-Beatty J.E., González-Rivera, M.D., Graupera, J.L., Martín, M., Campos, A., & Del Hierro, D. (2009). Los hábitos de actividad física de las mujeres mayores en España. *Revista Internacional de Ciencias del Deporte. 14* (5), 81–93.

Martínez, J., Jiménez-Beatty, J.E., Graupera, J.L., Martín, M., Campos, A. & Del Hierro, D. (2010). Being physically active in old age: Relationships with being active earlier in life, social status and agents of socialization. *Aging & Society, 30* (7), 1097–1113.

Martínez, J., Jiménez-Beatty, J.E., Santacruz, J.A., Martín, M., & Rivero, A. (2011). La recomendación médica y el tipo de demanda de actividad física en las personas mayores de la provincia de Guadalajara. *Revista Internacional de Ciencias del Deporte, 23* (7), 92–102.

Ministry of Health and Consumer Affairs (2005). *Estrategia para la Nutrición, Actividad Física y Prevención de la Obesidad (Estrategia NAOS)*. Madrid: Ministry of Health and Consumer Affairs.

Ministry of Health, Social Services and Equality (2014). *Estrategia de promoción de la salud y prevención en el Sistema Nacional de Salud. Informes, estudios e investigación 2014*. Madrid: Ministry of Health, Social Services and Equality. Retrieved from www.msssi.gob.es/profesionales/saludPublica/prevPromocion/docs/EstrategiaPromocionSaludyPrevencionSNS.pdf.

Ministry of Health, Social Services and Equality (n.d.). *Spanish national health survey 2011/12*. Retrieved from www.msssi.gob.es/estadEstudios/estadisticas/encuestaNacional/encuestaNac2011/encuestaResDetall2011.htm.

Moscoso, D., Moyano, E., Biedma, L., Fernández-Ballesteros, R., Martín, M., Ramos, C., & Serrano, R. (2009). *Deporte, salud y calidad de vida. Colección estudios sociales 26*, Barcelona: Fundación "La Caixa."

National Sports Council (NSC) (2009). *Comprehensive plan for physical activity and sport. Older adults V1*. Madrid: NSC.

National Sports Council (NSC) (2010). *Comprehensive Plan for Physical Activity and Sport*. Madrid: NSC.

National Sports Council (NSC) (2015). *Encuesta de hábitos deportivos en España 2015*. Madrid: Ministerio de Educación, Cultura y Deporte.

Pont, P. & Soler, A. (2011). La actividad física. In P. Causapié, A. Balbontín, M. Porras, & A. Mateo (Coords.), *Envejecimiento activo. Libro Blanco* (pp. 267–277). Madrid: Ministry of Health, Social Policy and Equality.

Romo-Pérez, V., Schwingel, A., & Chodzko-Zajko, W. (2011). International resistance training recommendations for older adults: Implications for the promotion of healthy aging in Spain. *Journal of Human Sport & Exercise, 6* (4), 369–648.

Salinas, F., Cocca, A., Mohamed, K., & Viciana, J. (2010). Actividad física y sedentarismo: Repercusiones sobre la salud y calidad de vida de las personas mayores. *Retos. Nuevas tendencias en educación física, Deporte y Recreación, 17*, 126–129.

Spanish National Institute of Statistics (2016). *España en cifras 2016*. Retrieved from www.ine.es/prodyser/espa_cifras.

Chapter 9

Physical activity, health, and body image of older adults in the Czech Republic

Ludmila Fialova

Introduction

The aim of this chapter is to understand the situation of seniors and the type of physical activities offered in the Czech Republic. After introducing the Czech Republic, the health status and demographic development in the country are clarified, followed by a description of the importance of physical activities for seniors. This chapter also deals with the benefits of physical activity for self- concept and body image. The number of Czech seniors participating in physical activities is addressed as well as recommendations for suitable activities for this population group.

The Czech Republic is a unitary parliamentary republic in Central Europe, with 10.5 million inhabitants. The capital and largest city is Prague, with over 1.2 million residents. The Czech State was formed in the late ninth century as the Duchy of Bohemia under the Great Moravian Empire. The kingdom of Bohemia was a significant regional power during the middle ages. Its greatest heyday was in the fourteenth century under the reign of the Czech king and Roman Caesar Charles IV. The Czech lands were under Habsburg rule from 1526, later becoming part of the Austrian empire and Austria- Hungary. The independent Republic of Czechoslovakia was established in 1918 after World War I. The Czech part of Czechoslovakia was occupied by Germany in World War II, and was liberated in 1945 by the armies of the Soviet Union and the United States. In 1989 with the Velvet Revolution, the communist regime collapsed and a multiparty parliamentary republic was formed. Czechoslovakia peacefully dissolved in 1993, with its constituent states becoming the independent states of the Czech Republic and Slovakia. The Czech Republic joined the North Atlantic Treaty Organization (NATO) in 1999, the European Union (EU) in 2004, and is a member of the United Nations, the Organization for Economic Co-operatio n and Development (OECD), the Organization for Security and Co-operation in Europe (OSCE), and the Council of Europe.

Health and demographic situation in the Czech Republic

According to the *National report about health* (Zprava o zdravi obyvatel Ceske Republiky, 2014) cardiovascular diseases have been the most common causes of death in the Czech Republic in the long term, killing 50 percent of the population. During the last decade, the mortality rate has been reduced by 20 percent, mainly due to more effective diagnostic and therapeutic procedures. In comparison to more developed EU countries, the mortality rate due to cardiovascular disease is twice as high in the Czech Republic.

Cancer is the second leading cause of death for both males and females. Severe diseases with high growth dynamics include diabetes mellitus (diabetes—Type 2). Allergic diseases represent a significant burden for public health. Asthma has become one of the most common chronic non-infectious diseases over the past few decades. The main reason for cardio-vascular disease and the increase of diabetes mellitus (Type 2) is based on the unhealthy life style of the Czech population. Physical activity is seldom part of a typical working day for the majority of Czech citizens, but unhealthy eating habits continue. The main reason for overweight is the high-energy intake through food and drinks, and low-energy expenditure through physical activity. Especially the older population (50+) is developing a lack of movement and physical activity. The membership in sport clubs for men is about 15 percent and for women less than 5 percent. This is quite surprising because in the Czech Republic 9-year-old children participate at a very high rate (girls: 35 percent, boys: 55 percent), and even 25 percent of 20-year-old men and women (almost same rate), participate in sport clubs (Rychtecký, 2006).

Furthermore, unhealthy food is typical in the Czech kitchen (food containing many carbohydrates, such as cakes, pies, dumplings) and the use of tobacco products are among the most significant risk factors, resulting in severe diseases and premature deaths. This could be avoided effectively through prevention. The Czech Republic is ranked first among all countries in Europe for the consumption of pure alcohol. High tolerance to alcohol consumption and the use of non-alcoholic drugs, including cannabis, prevails in Czech society, especially among young people.

Overweight individuals and obesity present major challenges for a significant number of Czechs. More than half of the adult population in the Czech Republic (57 percent) are overweight, and this number is difficult to reduce. Older men make up the highest proportion of overweight and obese members of the population. The main reason for being overweight is the high-energy intake through food and low-energy expenditure through physical activity. Unfortunately, the older population becomes inactive and many stop exercising, particularly in organized sports (WHO, 2015).

The healthy life expectancy of the population in the Czech Republic was estimated at 62 years in 2010, which is close to the EU average. Since 1962, this value has not grown and with an increase in life expectancy, an increasing number of years now are spent in poor health. There are, however, numerous countries where the situation is much more favorable. In Sweden, for example, the healthy life expectancy has increased by 9 years—up to 71—over the same period, which is 9 years more than in the Czech Republic. The percentage of people who are not self-sufficient is increasing proportionally with age, and nearly 30 percent of people over 80 are dependent on outside care today.

Looking at the demographic situation it must be mentioned that the number of seniors is increasingly rising and, according to scientific forecasts, people over 60 years of age will account for up to one-third of the population in the Czech Republic. People over 74 will make up one-quarter of the population in 2030 (Health 2020, 2014). The retirement age has been continuously increasing as well. According to government regulation, it is currently 66 years for men and 65 for women. In the time of socialism, a woman with two children retired at age 56, now (2015) at 60 and, in a few years, at 65, because the retirement age is extended by several months every year.

The Czech Republic ranks among countries with an increasing aging population. The causes of demographic aging are the growth of education and qualifications of the population, changes in the upbringing of children, changes in the lifestyle of the population, and the population migration from rural to urban areas. In 2011, there were 16 percent seniors in society (citizens aged 65+), while at the end of 2015 there were 18 percent. Considering the percentage of the overall population, the Czech Republic is placed in the second half of the imaginary table of all European countries.

The number of employed Czech men and women over 65 years of age has risen by almost one-third compared to 1995. Most seniors occupy managerial or highly specialized positions. Compared to previous years, the number of those who made money on the side in physically more demanding professions (e.g., craftsmen, machine operators) has diminished. The employment rate in the age group of 70–74 is the third highest in Europe (Jaroševský, 2016).

The poverty of senior women is a major challenge in the Czech Republic. Czech female pensioners, on average, receive one-fifth lower pension than their male counterparts. Women live longer; they often remain without a partner, and bear all the living expenses by themselves (MF DNES, 2016). Women in the Czech Republic earn almost a quarter less than men; therefore, they contribute less. This is because they work in sectors and professions with lower incomes. Even in the same positions, according to surveys, they tend to have lower incomes than their male colleagues. Because of lower pensions, women in old age are far more

susceptible to poverty than men. Sociologists refer to this as the feminiza-
tion of poverty (MF DNES, 2013). According to a report on gender equality undertaken by the government, nine out of ten poor people over 65
years of age in the Czech Republic are women. Thus, the Czech Republic
is the country with the highest proportion of senior women living in
poverty in Europe.

The impact of physical activity on seniors

The status of seniors in society is based on its relationship to others and
relates to changing roles, lifestyle, and economic security. Especially relo-
cation to a retirement home, hospital, or other facility, where elderly
persons lose privacy and homes, may lead to a serious social change. By
retiring, individuals lose their value in the labor market and perceived
social status. The significant impact of retiring from a job results in
changes in the economic well-being of elderly people, which often limits
them in their deeply rooted cultural and social activities. The consequences
of biological changes are also manifested in the social sphere. Declining
physical strength and deteriorating functions of the senses lead to necessary dependence on other people, and entails some psychological impacts.
All these changes can be impacted further by diseases, family problems,
loneliness, lack of finances, poor housing, and more. Therefore, it is
important that the elderly stay socially and physically active to combat
some of these changes and prolong their own decline.

The importance of physical activity for promoting health stems from the
fact that movement is one of the essential needs of human beings. Apart
from the quality of life, the very existence of humans in the biological sense
is related to movement. If an individual has insufficient locomotion, the
basic physiological processes are not sufficiently stimulated and this is negatively manifested in various disorders and diseases. The current conviction of the EU is that spending active leisure time by practicing sporting
activities has a significant positive influence on a person's socialization
and integration into society. Retired individuals who are having great
problems relating to the loss of their social status, can maintain it through
participation in sport and physical activity. Therefore, motor activity plays,
and will keep playing, a significant role in the quality of human life by creating and supporting the health of individuals and the above-mentioned
socialization.

There are, however, multiple obstacles to this goal, not only health-
related ones. This is the reason why many seniors are unable to do a
workout or perform some exercises due to fatigue or other health-related
problems. For seniors, it is very difficult to overcome habits, but exercise is
a habit that will keep people active. If previous locomotion and activities
are continued with an appropriate intensity, this will help to break the

negative habits and replace them with positive ones. Early incorporation of exercises into everyday life makes it easier to continue with it even in older age, when older people have more difficulty with new exercises. These, in turn, should be easier to understand, so as not to discourage them by the complexity or a fear of injury. It is necessary to set short-term goals and reasonable objectives and not to fix one's mind on long-term benefits only. It is particularly important to exercise in a group that will help to maintain resolution and regularity (Pelikan & Charvat, 2014).

On the other hand, data from casualty wards suggest that the number of older people who became injured during sport and exercise participation has been on the rise. A typical patient is a man or woman between 60 and 70 who has suffered a medium to serious injury while riding a bike, skiing, or hiking. This used to be a rare phenomenon in the past as this age category used to be treated exclusively for joint disorders, pains during walking, and similar ailments. Active seniors who are trying not to compromise their standard of living even in their eighties are an increasingly more frequent phenomenon. They do not want to give up their favorite activities or sport.

Very important is the motivation for sport activities. Slepicka, Mudrak, and Slepickova (2015) administered the sample to 388 older adults (aged 60+). Fifty-two percent stated that they participated in physical activity on a level recommended by the World Health Organization (WHO), 75 percent reported that they did not participate in any intensive physical activity, and 35 percent did not participate in moderate physical activity. The types of physical activity these seniors participated in where mainly gardening, working around the household, walking, dancing, swimming, or biking. Long-term participation in sports can modify the value orientations of older adults. Personal values may influence active participation in sports, the experience and the results of this participation, especially when the values are positively oriented toward sports. Value orientations may, therefore, support physically active lifestyles of the senior population.

Regular physical activity is associated with numerous health benefits, including reduced risks of cardiovascular disease, some types of cancer (e.g., breast, colon) and diabetes (Type 2). It also helps to maintain optimum body weight, improves the blood lipid profile, digestive tract function, and mental health (reduced stress, increased self-esteem and self-control, and the ability to concentrate) and boosts the body's immune system. Physical activity also helps to control existing health problems (e.g., Type 2 diabetes, high blood pressure, or high cholesterol levels), and it is also important for maintaining physical, mental, and cognitive health in older age. There is a link between physical activity and life expectancy, whereas physically active people tend to live longer than inactive ones. Insufficient physical activity along with poor eating habits leads to an increase in obesity in the population (Štilec, 2004).

Benefits of sport for self-concept and body image

Self-concept, a person's view of her- or himself, means more than just the opinions one has about the self. It also describes the relationship to one's self, including emotional experiences with cognitive, active, and regulative factors. The self is formed on a basic level of evaluation and becomes the object of opinions and attitudes. Research into self-concept has recently entered the area of sports and the physical self. A number of studies have been performed to determine what role physical aspects play in our overall self-concept. The physical self is believed to be a motivating agent of our behavior, significantly contributing to our overall self-respect, mental health, and well-being. The physical self-concept has been associated with sports or regular exercise that aims at keeping fit, achieving ideal weight, maintaining a healthy lifestyle, and the physical condition or rehabilitation after an injury or due to a disability. One may assume that regular physical activity may teach new skills to individuals and improve their physical fitness and health, thereby increasing their overall self-concept and self-respect. There are many models that describe the relationship between sport and self-concept.

Mudrak, Stochl, Slepicka, and Elavsky (2016) monitored 700 older Czech adults (aged ≥60 years) from all regions of the Czech Republic. The average age of the participants was 68 years of age (SD = 6.26). They found that increased participation in physical activities was associated with greater self-efficacy, which improved the mental and physical health status. In turn, self-efficacy and physical and mental health status were positively related to the overall quality of life, represented by the respondents' satisfaction with life. As hypothesized by the social cognitive theory (Bandura 1997), mastery of physical activities helps older people feel physically more in control of their bodies, which may translate into more positive evaluations of their health and also directly influence their satisfaction with life.

Compared to older Western adults (Bauman et al. 2008), Czech elderly who have not been physically active in the past may have less access to other sources of self-efficacy because they may lack opportunities to obtain social support and encouragement toward physical activities from their peers, as well as appropriate models providing vicarious experiences in their age group. Compared to older Western adults, older people from post-communist countries, generally, live in poorer socioeconomic conditions, adhere to behavioral norms that are less beneficial for their health, and perceive that they have less control over their health (Bobak et al. 2000; Carlson 1998; Dragomirecka et al. 2008; Eikemo et al. 2008; Laaksonen et al. 2001; Vuorisalmi et al. 2008). Bandura (1997) hypothesized that self-efficacy positively affects various aspects of life, including health, by facilitating "the exercise of control." In this way, people with high self-efficacy have an increased perception of themselves as agents of their own health, which allows them to actively engage in positive health-related behavior. However, self-efficacy might be less effective in older adults from post-communist countries, including the Czech Republic, as they seem to have (and perceive themselves to have) fewer opportunities to exercise their agency and positively influence their health by their own activity. The weaker mediating effect of health status may also partially result in the choice of physical activity in which the older Czech adults participate. It has been observed that older Czech adults participate in few physical leisure activities, preferring to participate in work-related physical activities (Laaksonen et al. 2001; Mudrak et al. 2012; Vohralikova & Rabusic, 2004).

Taking care of one's body and health has become a standard part of modern life. While our grandparents were happy just being healthy enough to bear and bring up children, our parents' generation is spending more and more effort and money in keeping up one's health, and looking good and being fit. Our children will face the risk of damaging both their bodies and minds with drastic diets, taking food supplements designed to increase muscle mass, undergoing plastic surgeries, and getting tattoos and piercings. Why is physical perfection so important to us, and why do we refuse to accept our natural selves? Psychologists and sociologists have spent years researching people's attitudes to themselves, including the very important issue of physical self-image. On one hand, lack of natural physical activity leads to growing masses of obese and ill individuals. On the other hand, we have seen a rise of eating disorders and other unfortunate practices that seriously damage the human body. There is no doubt that sufficient and appropriate physical activity should be included in the lifestyles of people of all ages as it represents one of most important factors of active and healthy aging (Ackni plan, 2016).

Body image is understood to be a complexity of all imaginations that are related to the human body. Therefore, it is characterized by cognitive (knowledge, convictions), effective (evaluation, self-confidence), and behavioral (self-control) components. Appearance and functionality of our body basically influences our physical and psychological condition and our behavior. The relationship to the body develops and changes during the lifespan. It is influenced by gender, age, sometimes by education, standard values, or physical activities (Fialova, 2001).

We observed and analyzed the relationship to the body, not as independent aspects of individual lifestyles but as components of the basic body concept (Fialova 2008, 2014, 2015; Fialova & Mrazek, 2005). Physical satisfaction is the result of individual experiences linked to one's own body and in many dimensions, it can be determined by the social environment. There is a large amount of information about sport activities and their influence on one's health, but little is known about the area of intentional, planned behavior, which contributes to one's personal satisfaction.

The subjective mental representations about one's body are very important for a positive change in the health behavior—changes in physical activity, nutrition, and health habits.

Physical activity influences the body image especially among adults. Fialova (2015) analyzed physical self in more than 800 adults aged 55+. Significant differences were found in the behavior and in the relationship to the body between physically active and less active people: people who are active in sports are more content with their appearance, shape, and their weight than less active people. The evaluation of all aspects of their body image is more positive, especially appearance and shape. Those who participate in sport in their leisure time, take greater care of their health, appearance, and shape. Mostly, active people are very interested in controlling their fitness. They also pay intense attention to their health, body, weight, and performance; they smoke less and spend more time outdoors. They also want to be more attractive to the other sex.

Men are significantly more satisfied with their shape, appearance, weight, and height, despite not paying attention to their appearance; however, they care more about their efficiency. Men evaluate their own fitness at a higher level than women, and, similarly, their appearance, but men's state of health is rated as worse than women's. Women admitted more often to headaches. In other areas, no significant differences were expressed between men and women. Both groups often admitted to back-aches and, less often, to heart complaints.

These results indicate that physical self-concept is largely determined by the gender of the person rather than other circumstances. Like other researchers (Fox 1990; Grogan 2000; Higgins et al. 1997), Fialova (2015) found that self-image and the attitude one takes to one's self and one's body depends primarily on the degree of physical activity and less on age, education, and other factors. The physically more active group appreciates the body and health more, and they are also significantly happier with the monitored aspects of their physical and mental state. At the same time, they feel more in control of their body and feelings. Active females tend to see more opportunity for change, which indicates a higher level of self-confidence. Furthermore, the number of health complaints reported by these respondents is significantly lower than those reported by inactive persons.

A surprising finding was that women declared greater importance of psychological aspects (thoughts and feelings) than of the physical aspects (body and health). This might be influenced by stress, work overload, tension, and worries that are part of everyday life. The importance of mental and physical health was recognized by more than 80 percent of women. In terms of psychological aspects, the most important factors were: life without fear and tension, independence of thought and action, feeling positive about self. In terms of physical aspects, the most important factors were hygiene, body care, and health. Physical activity and fitness were considered more important than looks and nutrition. In psychological terms, women were less satisfied in terms of a life free of tension and worries and the way they feel and think about themselves. Of the physical aspects, the least satisfactory physical aspects for women were activity and fitness and looks and nutrition. This dissatisfaction may lead women to adopt behavior that is commendable in terms of health but they may lack understanding and be susceptible to media pressure. Once the promised results fail to materialize, even more dissatisfaction may be felt. Women are considered more susceptible to advertising than men and many companies take clever advantage of this fact.

It was also found that those adults who do not participate in sport in their free time suffered more often from psychosomatic difficulties, including restless sleep, weariness, digestive problems, headaches, and backaches. This group is less satisfied with their health in comparison with the more active individuals and they consider their health as being poorer. Other results concerning satisfaction with their body (appearance, functioning, and fitness) as well as their relationship with their body suggests that the sporting population is more satisfied with their body image and is better able to cope with difficulties. In active seniors the psychic health and feeling of well-being is rated higher than in seniors with passive leisure programs.

Senior participation in physical activity in the Czech Republic

In general, older Czech adults may be characterized by a low preference for organized physical activity, low participation in sport and sport clubs, and high participation in non-sporting physical activities (Mudrak et al., 2012; Vohralikova & Rabusic, 2004). It has been reported that older Czech adults participate in sport organizations significantly less than their Western counterparts (Laaksonen et al., 2001; Vuorisalmi et al., 2008) with only 12 percent of older Czech adults participating in sports or exercise activities. On the other hand, 70 percent of Czech retirees aimed to improve their life by participating in the work-related physical activities that provide them and their families with additional sources of income and other benefits (Vohralikova & Rabusic, 2004).

EU comparison of physical activities in seniors

Recent data on the participation in sport and physical activity has been provided by EUROBAROMETR 412 (Slepicka et al., 2015). This study found that, in the EU, 48 percent of people participated in some type of physical activity at least once a week, while 30 percent did not participate in any physical activity. The level of physical activity decreases with age—71 percent of men and 70 percent of women aged 55 or older rarely or never participated in sport. People who participated in sports only rarely or never were, generally, people without paid work (72 percent of pensioners and 63 percent of unemployed). On average, just 30 percent of Europeans, aged 55+, participated in sports at least once a week, suggesting that relatively few European older adults managed to exercise at the recommended levels of physical activity. Non-sporting physical activity can also enrich people's lives and positively influence their health. Approximately 15 percent of EU citizens participate in non-sporting physical activity (such as cycling, dancing, or gardening) five times or more per week. Approximately one-third of EU citizens participate in this type of physical activity one to four times per week that implies that nearly half of EU citizens do not participate in this type of physical activity (Slepička et al., 2015).

Cultural differences have also been observed between various EU countries, particularly between the Nordic countries and others. For example, 31 percent of Finnish and Swedish adults and only 6 percent of Bulgarian and Polish adults report that they participate in sports for health-related reasons. It is approximately 14 percent in the Czech Republic, which suggests that there is relatively low awareness of the importance of physical activity for health among Czech adults. The situation in the Czech Republic can be illustrated further by the barriers the Czech adults mention in relation to their sporting physical activity. More than a half of them reported a lack of time as the most important barrier to physical activity. At the same time, in comparison with Nordic and other Western countries, the Czech adults spent more time sitting and watching TV. Researchers show that Czech pensioners tend to be more passive in their leisure time activities (Mudrak et al., 2016). It has been found that Czech pensioners spend, on average, 3 hours a day watching television during the week, and 3.5 hours per day during the weekends. This may stem from the fact that older Czech adults tend to spend their free time at home. It seems that their relatively low levels of sport participation and physical activity have been related to personal motivation rather than environmental factors, as the Czech seniors reported that they are physically active in parks, nature, and public spaces. Furthermore, 75 percent of Europeans and 96 percent of Czechs considered the conditions for access to sports in their neighborhoods as good.

Czech sports organization with a large seniors' membership base

The Czech Sokol (Falcon) Organization (Česká obec sokolská, ČOS) is the oldest gymnastic organization, and was established 1862. In 2016 there were more than 1,000 regional organizations with approximately 157,000 members. Sokol focuses on a wide range of abilities and ages, from young children to seniors. More than 90,000 members are adults (men: 45,200, women: 45,500) (Sokol, 2016). As in the past, ČOS aims its activities mainly on *sport for all*. This organization provides 56 different kinds of physical activities. Most of the members exercise in the Department of "General Development" contributing to general education. It offers an ideal opportunity to exercise with a group of seniors and perform regular physical activity. Sokol Festivals have a long tradition (beginning in 1882 with 720 gymnasts and 3,420 spectators), introducing mass public performances by Sokol members. In 2012, gymnasts of all age categories performed in mass demonstrations at the XV Sokol Festival in Prague. In the program were demonstrations for seniors (senior men and women together with "faithful guard") as well as adults. The XVI Sokol Festival will be held in 2018, but the preparation begins years earlier. In 2016 during the public performance, seniors performed their composition for the year 2018 with the name "Princess Republic" (the Czechoslovak Republic was founded 1918).

The Czech Association of Tourism (Český klub turistů, ČKT) is a famous institution with a long nationwide tradition dating back to the nineteenth century. Sport is provided especially for the older age category. There are nearly 650 clubs with more than 41,000 members. The most popular activity is an organized walking trip, where older adults participate. The excellent net (40,000 km) of well-marked and well-connected Czech hiking trails is the legacy of the work of ČKT. Today the hiking trails are still maintained by Czech Tourist Club members on a voluntary basis. Signposts at main hiking route junctions also include kilometers to the nearest towns (Klub českých turistů, 2016).

The Czech Association Sport for All (CASPV) offers various choices of movement activities: general gymnastics, recreational sports, aerobics, rhythmical gymnastics, yoga, heath-oriented exercises, psychomotor, nature exercises, dancing, traditional Chinese exercise, etc. There are more than 60,000 registered members and more than 40,000 in associated subjects (the majority are adults and seniors) (Ceska Asociace Sport pro Vsechny, 2016).

Part of the senior population regularly or sporadically participates in Seniors' sport (Sport seniorů, 2016) for physical activities and sport. In 2016, numerous sports competitions were organized from club events via mini-regional and municipal events to district, national, and international events. Among dozens of organized competitions there are, e.g., the Municipal Sports Games in Ostrava. The seniors of Ostrava performed multidisciplinary events (e.g., penalty free throws in basketball, throwing darts, ball throw at cans, and tennis skills). Slovak seniors were also invited to regional sport games. Nearly 200 athletes participated in the regional sports games. The program consisted of individual competitions in senior multidiscipline events and a tournament of teams in a ringo game in the sand. Subsequently, Czech seniors accepted the invitation to participate in the Slovak National Games. The culmination of seniors' efforts was Prague International Sports Games with the participation of 25 eight-member teams from the whole country and some Slovak regions.

Sanatoria for long-term ill people (stay up to 3 months) provide physiotherapists who organize exercises for patients several times a week. This includes old people's homes, where the average age is over 80, with exercise for those interested being offered twice a week in a specially designated activity room. In modern institutions, walking tours and outdoor fitness centers (simple exercise machines) are offered, usually in gardens.

Conclusion

It can be stated that physical activities for seniors can help to reduce the sickness rate and allows being active. Regular physical activity has been proven to have a positive effect on cardiovascular diseases, diabetes mellitus (Type 2), osteoporosis, arthritis, urination difficulties, development of cancer, obesity, and others. Exercising assists depression, supports the extension of social contacts, improves the ability to learn, especially short-term memory, and influences the quality of sleep. Physical activity improves self-concept, self-satisfaction, self-confidence, and self-efficacy.

There is still a lack of research in the field of behavioral health and aging in the Czech Republic. In the future, experts should focus on the possibilities of increasing physical activity, decreasing sedentary life styles, and improving the health status, especially for the older population. To be vital in advanced age, health, and varied alimentation, a positive attitude to life and regular enjoyable physical activity is very important. The worst influences are sitting watching television and using the computer, together with the consumption of unhealthy food and general passivity. For older people, the goal should primarily be living longer in the best mental and physical condition as possible, including meaningful physical activity.

Recommendations

Physical activity should be an important concern of public health programs in countries where the trend toward "active aging" has emerged only recently, such as in post-communist countries in general, and in the Czech Republic in particular (Bauman et al. 2008). Such interventions should focus on the development of self-efficacy as an important predictor of future physical activity habits and should recognize that reduced self-efficacy may lead to a decrease in both sport participation and the quality of life of older adults (Warner et al., 2011). The interventions should include a focus on lifelong participation in physical activities because the most efficient method of developing self-efficacy is to master activities, and self-efficacy of older adults may stem from their physical activity participation at a younger age (Bandura, 1997). Interventions involving physical activity for leisure seem to be under-developed for older adults in the Czech Republic and other post-communist countries. The introduction of such timely interventions can provide important positive influences on health and the overall quality of life.

The aging population in the Czech Republic needs to prepare for active leisure time activities for seniors; for example, instructors' training, public facilities for these activities, diversity of activities offering, financial accessibility, prophylactic organized programs, and more. Only some seniors have participated in sport and physical activity their whole life, and are mostly in excellent health. They participate in a wide variety of physical activity, similar to people one generation younger. But there are also those seniors with health limitations, practicing little or no physical activity. It is necessary to stress to this group that exercising is essential for their quality of life, with a starting point for all ages. The difference between seniors' physical activities compared to younger ages is primarily in the slower pace because of the higher risk of vascular attacks in older people. The activity should not try to increase the heart rate as much as for younger sports' participants. It is necessary to eliminate exercises with the head downward and to perform position changes in slower motion. Physical activities twice a week and daily home activities aimed at flexibility are optimal. Regular physical activity can substantially slow the negative effects of aging. Active seniors have better postural habits with correct breathing, greater mobility, and suffer less pain. Physical activity is not only the base for body consolidation; it also influences spirit and self-confidence. Active people feel more energy and spend more time joyfully, relaxing and having less depression and anxiety. They are seldom hypochondriacs, have better sleeping patterns, and enhanced digestion. They have fewer body problems and at lower risk of heart disease and strokes. Active people have stronger bones, toned bodies, better weight control, and find that going about their daily tasks is easier.

These types of physical activities are beneficial for seniors:

Aerobic exercise has a very positive influence, especially on the cardiovascular and respiratory systems. Activities in this category may include:

- Tourism, above all Nordic walking (with special sticks, involving up to 90 percent of muscles) helps to improve heartbeat, supplying the organs with oxygen and improving metabolism. Walking improves postural habits, helping to prevent backache. Even going for a walk encourages physical fitness. Seniors can mix slow walking with the faster, trying the "Indian run."

- Swimming and aqua gymnastics are ideal activities for seniors. Weight is evenly spread and stretches the whole body. The water raises the body, saving wear and tear on the joints, vertebral column, and ligaments. Swimming is particularly suitable for people who are overweight or obese. Furthermore, swimming strengthens the cardiovascular system and improves heart activity, supports the respiratory system, tones muscles, and increases mobility and balance ability. Swimming has a positive effect on muscular tension and the psyche.

- Cross-country skiing stretches and works up to 90 percent of the body's muscle system. The muscles in the arms and legs work equally, as do the deep core muscles surrounding the spine because it is necessary during skiing to maintain balance. Cross-country skiing improves the cardiovascular system and spinal posture. Seniors can cross-country ski in winter on snow everywhere in the safe terrain of parks and the countryside.

- Cycling is especially appropriate for seniors, because, unlike walking or running, it does not create pressure on joints. Therefore, it is suitable for people rehabilitating after joint disease. It assists obese people to lose weight. Researchers have stated that regular biking improves the physical condition of seniors so it is comparable with people 10 years younger. It is also an effective prophylaxis of coronary occlusion, raised blood pressure, embolism, and stroke. It was shown that cycling helps to decrease eye-pressure, which is the highest risk of glaucoma and occurs particularly in the older age group. Biking is possible everywhere, in the city or using a stationary bike at home. There are hundreds of kilometers of new bike pathways in the Czech Republic.

- Dancing, or simple steps to music, rhythmic exercises, or creative movements to music are suitable exercises, used not only as a warm up, but also involving individuals in a social group; dancing can also be practiced in pairs. These activities not only bring joy, but also support memory, coordination, and spatial orientation functions.

Weight training: Working out is very important for older people to prevent muscles weakening and bones becoming less dense. Fitness exercises improve body posture, range of movement, muscle strength, and coordination. They develop feelings of self-satisfaction and self-confidence. Fitness centers offer exercises for seniors in their programs and also employ specialists in exercises tailored for seniors. Strengthening the skeletal muscles is especially important in old age. One must distinguish between the type of training involved—advanced or beginner. Exercises involving the body being upside down, and exercises using excessive weight or frequent changes in positions should be avoided. The workout in the gym should finish with stretching. It is possible to carry out the workout in the gym (fitness center), at home or outside. More than 100 projects of outside fitness were realized in the last year in the Czech Republic—within the purview of European year of active aging and generation solidarity. The point is the installation of outside exercise and massage machines allow seniors to exercise for free in fresh air. Seniors are not only working out, but also maintaining motor skills. The advantage is that the person uses their own body weight as the load during the exercise.

Coordination exercises: Exercise at home can be a great advantage, because seniors can participate at any time when they desire and have time to organize everything they need. It is also possible to visit the fitness center and consult with the trainer. Many fitness centers and local subdivisions of Sokol organize exercises directly for seniors, where the instructors takes account of their needs. Many exercises that seniors learn can be done alone at home, especially balance practice, improving self-sufficiency, rehabilitation, and health movements. Examples include:

- Relaxation and compensation exercises are vital for maintaining joint mobility, as well as alleviating the functional disorders of the locomotor system. It is noted that the technique of good posture, the practice of sitting, standing up, and walking, together with the compensation for muscle imbalance, have positive effects on seniors. Breathing and relaxation exercises develop an awareness of one's own body. Exercises enhancing fine motor skills, finger exercises in particular, must also be included.
- Psychomotor games are often popular in group exercises. In these games, the emphasis is mainly on the actual experience of locomotion. They do not require maximum strength, performance, or victory over others. The essence of psychomotorics is a game during which the participants get to know each other as well as get to know their body and the environment. Their communication with others is also enhanced. Another advantage is the elimination of inhibitions, stress, and fear.
- Exercises with Eastern philosophical orientation—yoga, tai chi, and chi gong have recently grown in popularity. Eastern medicine perceives humans in connection with the environment. Most of the Eastern exercises work with the energy that is inside each of us. They work with a positive attitude toward conducted exercises, breathing, and the awareness of one's own body. Concentration and patience are also important.
- Stretching draws out the muscles and reduces muscle tension after the physical load and keeps muscles flexible. It also prevents against back pain. The use of stretching is widely used, not only in sport, but also in medical rehabilitation. It attends to injury prophylaxis—preventing a muscle tear and inflammation of the tendons.

- Table tennis is an appropriate activity for seniors because it puts the whole body in motion and trains observation and motoric, as well as being enjoyable. According to experts, table tennis can prevent Alzheimer's. Table tennis is often offered free of charge at various clubs, in activity centers' programs for seniors, and even in homes for the elderly.

References

Akcni plan pohybove activity CR (2016, February 12). Retrieved from http://docplayer.cz/5354841-Akcni-plan-c-1-podpora-pohybove-aktivity-na-obdobi-2015-2020.html.

Bandura, A. (1997). *Self-efficacy. The exercise of control.* New York: Freeman.

Bauman, A., Schoeppe, S., & Lewicka, M. (2008). *Review of best practice in interventions to promote physical activity in developing countries.* Geneva: WHO.

Bobak, M., Pikhar, H., Rose, R., Hertzman, C., & Marmot, M. (2000). Socioeconomic factors, material inequalities, and perceived control in self-rated health: cross-sectional data from seven post-communist countries. *Social Science and Medicine, 51*, 1343–1350.

Carlson, P. (1998). Self-perceived health in East and West Europe: another European health divide. *Social Science and Medicine, 45*, 1355–1366.

Ceska Asociace Sport pro Všechny (2016, February 12). Retrieved from www.caspv.cz/cz/o-nas/zakladni-informace/.

ČSSZ (2016). Retrieved from https://eportal.cssz.cz/web/portal/tiskopisy-osvc-2016.

Dragomirecka, E., Bartonova, J., Eiseman, M., Kalfoss, M., Kilian, R., Martiny, K., von Steinbuchel, N., & Schmidt, S. (2008). Demographic and psychosocial correlates of quality of life in the elderly from a cross-cultural perspective. *Clinical Psychology and Psychotherapy, 15*, 193–204.

Eikemo, T., Bambra, C., Judge, K., & Ringdal, K. (2008). Welfare state regimes and differences in self-perceived health in Europe: a multilevel analysis. *Social Science and Medicine, 66*, 2281–2295.

Fialova, L. (2001). *Body image jako součást sebepojetí člověka.* Praha: Nakladatelství Karolinum.

Fialova, L. (2008). Stárnutí, vztah k tělu a životní styl žen ve věku nad 40 let. *Česká kinantropologie, 12*(3), 17–25.

Fialova, L. (2014). Differences in body image and health among sport active and passive adults as a base for school health education. *American Journal of Educational Research, 2*(9), 782–787.

Fialova, L. (2015). Personal satisfaction, physical self and health related behavior from the aspect of involvement in sports in adult population In: T. Louková, B. Hátlová, M. Adámková (Eds.), *Psychomotor therapy* (pp. 55–66). Ústí nad Labem: University of J. E. Purkyně.

Fialova, L. & Mrazek, J. (2005). Sportengagement und Körperkonzepte von Frauen. *Sport in Europa*, 212–213. Hamburg: Czwalina Verlag.

Fox, K. R. (1990). *The physical self-perception profile manual.* De Kalb, IL: Northern Illinois University Office for Health Promotion.

Grogan, S. (2000). *Body image, psychologie nespokojenosti s vlastním tělem.* Praha: Grada Publishing.

Health 2020 – National Strategy for Health Protection and Promotion and Disease Prevention. (2014). Praha: Ministry of Health of the Czech Republic.

Higgins, E., Shah, J., & Friedman, R. (1997). Emotional responses to goal attainment: strength of regulatory focus as moderator. *Journal of Personality and Social Psychology, 72,* 515–525.

Jaroševský, F. (2016). Stárneme jako Němci. *Metro,* October 19, 2016, 6.

Klub českých turistů (2016, May 4). Retrieved from www.kct.cz/cms/kalendar-turistickych-akci.

Laaksonen, M., McAlister, A., Laatikainen, T., Drygas, W., Morova, E., Nussel, E., Oganov, R., Pardell, H., Uhanov, M., & Puska, P. (2001). Do health behaviour and psychosocial risk factors explain the European East-West gap in health status? *European Journal of Public Health, 11,* 65–73.

MF DNES (2013, July 9). Ženy mají o pětinu hubenější důchod než muži, častěji jim hrozí chudoba. Retrieved from http://ekonomika.idnes.cz/zeny-maji-o-petinu-hubenejsi-duchod-nez-muzi-casteji-jim-hrozi-chudoba-1e5-/ekonomika.aspx?c=A130709 170236 ekonomika vem.

Ministry of Health (2016, March 8). Retrieved from www.mzcr.cz/.

Mudrak, J., Elavsky, S., & Slepicka, P. (2012) Physical activity and its social-cognitive correlates in Czech and American older adults. *Czech Kinanthropology, 16*(3), 49–63.

Mudrak, J., Stochl, J., Slepicka, P., & Elavsky, S. (2016). Physical activity, self-efficacy, and quality of life in older Czech adults. *European Journal of Aging, 13*(1), 5–14.

Pelikán, Š. & Charvát, P. (February 12, 2016). Senioři a pohybová aktivita. Retrieved from www.vemeste.cz/2011/05/seniori-a-pohybova-aktivita/.

Rychtecký, A. (2006). *Monitorování účasti mládeže ve sportu a pohybové aktivitě v České republice.* Monografie. Praha: Universita Karlova, Fakulta tělesné výchovy a sportu.

Slepicka, P., Mudrak, J., & Slepickova, I. (2015). *Sport a pohyb v životě seniorů.* Praha: Karolinum.

Slepickova, I. & Slepicka, P. (2004). Proměny organizovaného sportu v České republice na přelomu století v kontextu podpory zdraví. In R. Vobr (Ed.), *Tělesná výchova a zdraví II.* (pp. 104–108). České Budějovice: JU PedF.

Sokol. Cz – Informační portál (2016). Retrieved from https://sokol.cz/sokol/.

Spirduso, W. W. (1995). *Physical dimensions of aging.* Champaign, IL: Human Kinetics.

Sport seniorů, (2016, March 7). Retrieved from www.sportjm.cz/sportovni-den-senioru-lednice-2016.

Štilec, M. (2004). *Program aktivního života pro seniory.* Praha: Portál.

Vohralikova, L. & Rabusic, L. (2004). *Čeští senioři včera, dnes a zítra.* Brno: VUPSV.

Vuorisalmi, M., Pietila, I., Pohjolainen, P., & Jylha, M. (2008). Comparison of self-rated health in older people of St Petersburg, Russia, and Tampere, Finland: how sensitive is SRH to cross-cultural factors? *European Journal of Ageing, 5,* 327–334.

Warner, L. M., Schultz, B., Knittle, K., Ziegelmann, J. P., Wurm, S. (2011). Sources of perceived self-efficacy as predictors of physical activity in older adults. *Applied Psychology: Health and Wellbeing, 3,* 172–192.
WHO (2015, October 11). Retrieved from www.who.int/gho/publications/world_health_statistics/2015/en/.
Zpráva o zdraví obyvatel České republiky (2014, April 6). Retrieved from www.mzcr.cz/verejne/dokumenty/zprava-o-zdravi-obyvatel-ceske-republiky2014-_9420_3016_5.html.

Chapter 10

Active and fit while climbing the ladder of life

Physical activity in old age in the young country Israel

Yael Netz

Introduction—Israel's population

Israel's population stood at a record 8,680,000 in May 2017, on Independence Day. This is a ten-fold increase compared to the population when the State of Israel was founded in 1948. The Jewish population comprises 6,484,000 (74.7 percent); 1,808,000 (20.8 percent) are Arabs (Muslims, Christian-Arabs, and Druze); and other groups (non-Arab Christians, Baha'i, and persons not classified by religion) make up 4.5 percent of the population (388,000 people). When the state was established, there were only 806,000 residents, and the total population reached its first and second million in 1949 and 1958, respectively. Judging by current population trend data, experts predict that the population of Israel will reach 10 million by 2025 or sooner (Jewish Virtual Library, 2017). In 2012, together with Australia and Japan, Israel had the highest life expectancy at birth in the world for males—about 80 years. Life expectancy at birth in Israel for females was 84 years, fourth highest in the world (MASHAV Planning for the Elderly, 2015). Figure 10.1 shows the increase in life expectancy in Israel from 1975–2014.

When Israel was established, it was a young society, with just 4 percent of its population aged 65 and over. The first large immigration wave was composed mainly of European Jews, most of whom were young people who had survived World War II. The most recent wave of immigrants began in 1989 from the former Soviet Union. Since then, approximately 730,000 people have arrived in Israel, increasing its population by about 20 percent. The relatively high percentage of elderly people among them (16 percent) significantly increased the absolute number of elderly people in Israel, as well as their proportion in the general population (Israel Aging Population, 2017). Consequently, in 2014 for example, only 21 percent of elderly Jews were Israel-born, compared with 75 percent of the Jewish general population (MASHAV Planning for the Elderly, 2015).

In addition to the effect of immigration on Israel's demography, the percentage of the elderly population is also increasing due to a decrease in

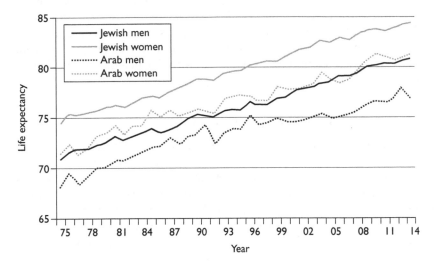

Figure 10.1 Life expectancy at birth in Israel by population group and gender, 1975–2014.

Source: Ministry of Health, Israel, Center for Disease Control (ICDC), Publication 371, Highlights of Health in Israel, 2016, www.health.gov.il/publicationsfiles/highlights_of_health_in_israel2016.pdf.

birth rate and increase in life expectancy. The percentage of people aged 65 and over grew from 4 percent in 1948 to 10.7 percent in 2014. The population of people aged 75 and over (the "old-old") has grown even more rapidly. Thus, not only has the general population been aging, but also the old population itself has been growing older. For example, by the end of 1998, the old-old group comprised 42.5 percent of people aged 65 and over. This trend is expected to continue. In 2020, elderly people will make up close to 12 percent of the general population, and the old-old will constitute about 50 percent of the total elderly population (Israel Aging Population, 2017). Even the group of 80 years or more is rapidly increasing. In 2014, 26 percent of the 65+ population were 80 years old or more, up from 14 percent in 1980 (MASHAV Planning for the Elderly, 2015).

Compared to the Organisation for Economic Co-operation and Development (OECD) countries, Israel's population is still relatively young. In 2014, 28.2 percent of the population of Israel were under age 15. In contrast, in the OECD countries this age group comprised 18.1 percent of the population. Conversely, the population of Israel aged 65 and above comprised 10.7 percent of the total population in 2014, as compared with 16.0 percent in the OECD countries. The Arab population in Israel is younger than the Jewish population: in 2014, 35.1 percent of the Arab population was under age 15, as compared to 26.4 percent of the Jewish population;

and 4.3 percent was aged 65 and over, as compared to 12.4 percent of the Jewish population (Ministry of Health, 2016). While life expectancy in Israel is one of the highest in the world, Israel is still considered a young country with about 11 percent people age 65 and above. Only 21 percent of elderly Jews are Israel-born, compared with 75 percent of the Jewish general population.

Physical activity in old age in Israel

Data on physical activity in Israel have been collected over the years as part of general health and health behavior surveys of various bodies, such as the Central Bureau of Statistics, and the Ministry of Health—the Centre of Disease Control and/or Department of Nutrition. The largest and most informative survey is probably the *Israeli National Health Interview Survey* (INHIS). This survey was developed within the framework of the World Health Organization (WHO), and has been conducted three times in Israel (2003–2004, 2007–2010, and 2014–2015). Each time the survey included 10,000 Israelis 21 years old and above—men, women, Jews, and Arabs. Based on the most updated information, 35.2 percent of respondents reported engaging in regular physical activity, 41.0 percent men and 29.6 percent women, according to the WHO recommendations: moderate physical activity for at least 150 minutes a week or intense activity for at least 75 minutes per week, or a combination of both. More specifically, by population group, 43.7 percent of Jewish men, 31.9 percent of Jewish women, 28.7 percent of Arab men, and 18.1 percent of Arab women reported physical activity in accordance with these recommendations (Ministry of Health, 2016).

Figure 10.2 presents the percentage of regular physical activity in Israel by age, gender, and population groups. Based on this figure, in the Jewish population physical activity rates in men were similar across all age groups, with the highest rate (45.2 percent) seen in those aged 35–49 years. In women, rates increased with age and reached 41.5 percent in those aged 65 years and above, compared with 21.0 percent in ages 21–34. In the Arab population, rates of physical activity decreased with age in both men and women; in men from 34.6 percent in ages 21–34 to 19.5 percent at age 65+, and in women from 23.5 percent in ages 21–34 to 5.6 percent at age 65+.

Several research projects have examined physical activity patterns of older adults in Israel in relation to demographic, health, and psycho-social aspects. All publications are based on large random samples of older adult Israelis; they include:

- Cohen-Mansfield and colleagues focused on national random samples of *older Jewish adults aged 75–94* (Cohen-Mansfield, 2012; Cohen-Mansfield & Kivity, 2011; Cohen-Mansfield, Shmotkin, & Goldberg, 2010);

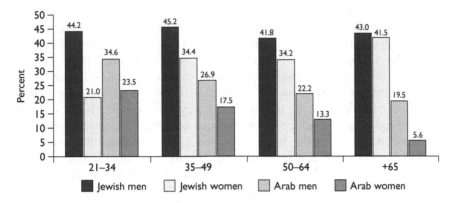

Figure 10.2 Regular physical activity* in Israel, by age, gender, and population group. INHIS-3, 2014–2015.

Source: Ministry of Health, Israel, Center for Disease Control (ICDC), Publication 371, Highlights of Health in Israel, 2016, www.health.gov.il/publicationsfiles/highlights_of_health_in_israel2016.pdf.

Note
* According to WHO Recommendations.

- Netz and colleagues analyzed a national random sample of both Jews and Arabs aged 65 and over (Dunsky et al., 2014; Netz, Dunsky et al., 2012; Netz, Goldsmith et al., 2012; Netz et al., 2011);
- The *Jerusalem Longitudinal Cohort Study* led by Stessman and colleagues, studied a representative sample of Jewish residents of Jerusalem aged 70 at baseline (Jacobs et al., 2013; Stessman & Jacobs, 2014; Stessman et al., 2000; Stessman et al., 2009); and
- an additional study focused on a national random sample of Jews and Arabs aged 60 and over was also reviewed (Litwin, 2003).

The following physical activity habits as related to demographic and health factors have been found among older Jewish Israelis aged 75–94. Cohen-Mansfield and colleagues studied the exercise behavior of older Jewish Israelis, aged 75–94 (Cohen-Mansfield, 2012; Cohen-Mansfield & Kivity, 2011; Cohen-Mansfield, Shmotkin, & Goldberg, 2010). The sample was randomly selected from the *Israel National Population Register*, a complete listing of the Israeli population maintained by the Ministry of the Interior. Physical activity was measured by the frequency of participation in five activities requiring physical effort. Furthermore, Cohen-Mansfield and her colleagues (2010) analyzed time changes in physical activity behavior among older adults.

The findings indicated that engagement in physical activity declined longitudinally. Physical activity was associated with good health and cognitive and mental functioning, suggesting that a decline in health and function impedes physical activity, or alternatively reduction in physical activity is responsible for the decline in health and function. In examining factors predicting the decline in physical activity along the years, the authors revealed that age (as people get older they are less active), gender (men are more active than women), and number of medications (more medications—less physical activity) were the strongest predictors of the decrease in frequency of physical activity. In examining factors predicting the initiation of physical activity, functional status and cognitive status were the best predictors. The interpretation was that cognitive resources might be needed to comply with and adhere to physical activity, as are the functional resources to enable the decision to participate.

Further studies by Cohen-Mansfield and her colleagues analyzed the initial wave of the data and an additional representative sample of same age cohort (age 75–94). In one study (Cohen-Mansfield & Kivity, 2011), it was indicated that physical activity and other common health behaviors (e.g., alcohol use, smoking, and nutrition) are unrelated. Thus, programs for promoting physical activity should be specific. The fact that data collection of the two cohorts was about 10 years apart (1989–1992 vs. 2000–2002) made it possible to compare the cohorts and examine changes in the patterns of physical activity over this period. Evidently, the findings suggest that the new cohorts of old-old persons are more physically active than the previous cohorts for the whole population, as well as for each gender (Cohen-Mansfield, 2012). Interestingly, the trend of increased activity in successive cohorts is contrary to the longitudinal trend evidenced in the previous study of Cohen-Mansfield and her colleagues following the same cohort of older adults age 75–94 (Cohen-Mansfield et al., 2010), which indicated a decline in physical activity. The explanation was that while older persons advance into old-old age their level of physical activity decreases, probably due to increased frailty and health problems, newer cohorts (successive cohorts) of old-old persons are in better health than previous cohorts and are probably more updated regarding the importance of physical activity.

The *Mabat Zahav Survey* represents a cross-sectional study by Netz and her colleagues (2011) looking at Jewish and Arab Israelis aged 65+. Although it did not report physical activity patterns in successive cohorts of older adults nor a longitudinal trend of physical activity in the same cohort, it was more inclusive in that it was comprised of a random sample of both Jewish and Arab older adult Israelis, and the age range of participants included persons 65 years old and over. Participants in that study were interviewed on their physical activity habits (data was collected in 2005–2006). The set of questions included type of activity, intensity, frequency, duration (months or years), and average length of their involvement. Based on the WHO recommendations, participants were divided into groups reflecting three levels of exercise:

(1) *sufficiently active* – those who were involved in moderate physical activity for at least 150 minutes a week or in intensive activity for at least 75 minutes per week, or a combination of the two; (2) *insufficiently active* – those who were involved in physical activity, but a lesser amount than the above; and (3) *inactive* – those who report no physical activity.

When health variables were examined as relating to the level of physical activity—not surprisingly and in agreement with the literature in all Western countries, dose-dependent relationships were revealed between Body Mass Index (BMI), functional level, chronic illness index, number of medications, and self-rated health, with the more favorable scores for the sufficiently active, followed by the insufficiently active and then the inactive (Netz et al., 2011).

Figures 10.3–10.8 present demographic information as related to level of physical activity (based on the *Mabat Zahav Survey*; Netz et al., 2011). Based on these figures, more men than women, more Jews than Arabs, and more secular than religious people (in both Jews and Arabs), were sufficiently active. In relation to birth origin, among both the Europe and US group and the Israeli-born group, the largest percentages were observed in the sufficiently active followed by the insufficiently active and the inactive,

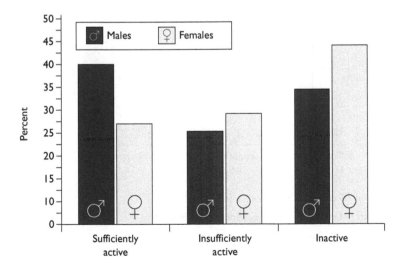

Figure 10.3 Level of physical activity by gender.

Source: Israel Ministry of Health, Mabat Zahav Survey, Netz et al., 2011.

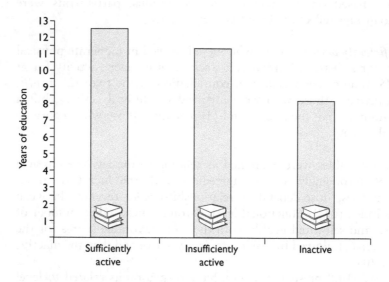

Figure 10.4 Level of physical activity by years of education.

Source: Israel Ministry of Health, Mabat Zahav Survey, Netz et al., 2011.

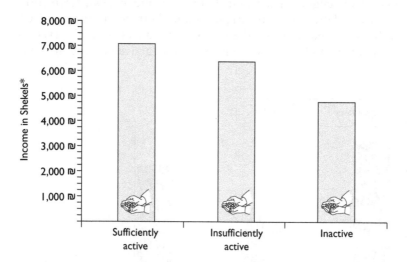

Figure 10.5 Level of physical activity by income.

Source: Israel Ministry of Health, Mabat Zahav Survey, Netz et al., 2011.

Note
* US$1 = 3.7 Israeli Shekels.

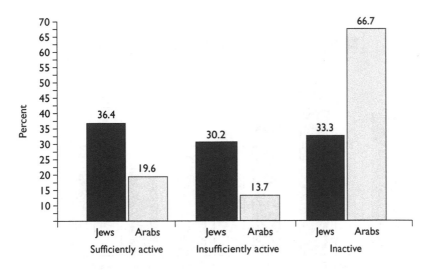

Figure 10.6 **Level of physical activity by population group.**

Source: Israel Ministry of Health, Mabat Zahav Survey, Netz et al., 2011.

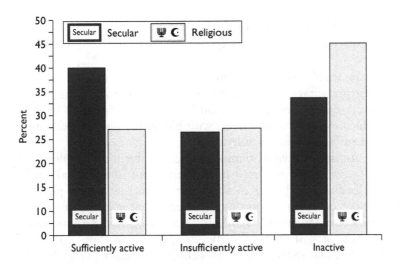

Figure 10.7 **Level of physical activity and religious vs. secular (in Jews and Arabs together).**

Source: Israel Ministry of Health, Mabat Zahav Survey, Netz et al., 2011.

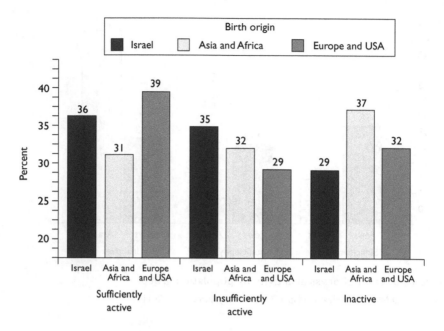

Figure 10.8 Level of physical activity by birth origin.

Source: Israel Ministry of Health, Mabat Zahav Survey, Netz et al., 2011.

while an opposite trend was observed among the Asian- and African-born, with the highest percentage in the inactive group. In support of the world-wide literature, a dose-dependent relationship appeared between level of activity and education and income level, with higher income and education observed in the sufficiently active individuals.

Similar relationships between demographic and health variables, and physical activity, were also reported in the Jerusalem longitudinal study, which is described in detail later in this chapter. In that study, physical activity was more common among participants from a European or US origin (as opposed to African or Asian), and was associated with increased years of education, lack of financial difficulties, less depression, good self-rated health status, and independence in activities of daily living. Physic-ally active participants took fewer medications and reported fewer falls or fractures and less chronic joint or musculoskeletal pain (Stessman et al. 2009).

In support of international publications (American College of Sports Medicine (ACSM), 2009), the most frequent physical activity reported in this study was walking (Litwin, 2003; Stessman et al., 2009). Table 10.1 presents the distribution of exercise type preferred by older adults in Israel (source: *Mabat Zahav*, Netz et al., 2011). Interestingly, the order of

Table 10.1 Types of activity in the sufficiently and insufficiently active older adults

	Insufficiently active		Sufficiently active	
	Average time in minutes (SD)	N (%)	Average time in minutes (SD)	N (%)
Walking	56.71 (26.80)	309 (68)	144.80 (90.73)	503 (91)
Light	43.05 (24.42)	189 (42)	74.04 (49.98)	199 (36)
Swimming	46.49 (25.07)	38 (8)	86.92 (71.41)	135 (24)
Body shaping	40.00 (0)	15 (7)	72.54 (57.32)	67 (23)
Cycling	37.39 (31.51)	23 (5)	62.06 (59.17)	71 (13)
Jogging	80.00 (0)	1 (0.5)	48.00 (23.48)	10 (4)

Source: Accepted author manuscript version reprinted, by permission, from *Journal of Aging and Physical Activity*, 2011, 19, 30–47, © 2011 Human Kinetics, Inc.

preferred activities was common to both sufficiently and insufficiently active individuals, with light exercise following walking, followed by swimming, body shaping, cycling, and jogging.

An interesting report based on the *Mabat Zahav Survey* informed about a relationship between level of physical activity and favorable anthropometric characteristics in older adults (Dunsky et al., 2014). Investigators found in both genders an association between level of physical activity and weight, waist circumference, and BMI, with lower values among the sufficiently active. In addition, a relationship between level of physical activity and height was indicated among women, implying that the more active women were taller than the less active.

Summarizing the key findings of the research on physical activity among older people in Israel, the following association was found between physical activity and demographic data: More men than women, more Jews than Arabs, and more secular than religious people (in both Jews and Arabs) are sufficiently active, meaning they adhere to physical guidelines recommended by official organizations. Generally, men reported being more physically active than women in the Jewish population, among both the European- and US-born groups as well as the Israeli-born, while an opposite trend is reported among the Asian- and African-born. Walking is the physical activity most frequently reported. Trends in physical activity include: as people get older they are less active; and based on successive cohorts, there is an increase in physical activity in old age. Last, there is a clear association between health and physical activity: decline in physical activity is associated with decline in health; there is a dose-dependent relationship between physical activity and BMI, functional level, chronic illness, number of medications, and self-related healthy—all in favor of physical activity. The studies also found that physical activity and other health behavior, such as alcohol use, smoking, and nutrition, are not necessarily related.

Physical activity and social connectedness

Social connectedness and the relations to physical activity in old age were also studied (Litwin, 2003; Netz, Goldsmith et al., 2012). Physical activity in the Litwin study (2003) was determined on the basis of a global dichotomous question: "Do you engage in physical activity on a regular basis?" to which respondents replied simply "yes" or "no." In the Netz et al. study (2012), three levels of physical activity were determined based on official recommendations (as explained above): sufficiently active, insufficiently active, and inactive.

Social connectedness in the Litwin study (2003) was based on five social networks into which the participants were grouped: the diverse-network, the friends-network, the neighbors-network, the family-network, and the restricted-network. The diverse-network was considered the most comprehensive social network in terms of the range of sources of contacts and potential support present in this group. When compared with respondents in the diverse-network, those in all the other network types had a significantly lower likelihood of reporting physical activity. Respondents categorized in a friends-network or a neighbors-network in this study were less likely than respondents in the diverse-network to report physical activity, and the family-network and restricted-network had the least chances to report physical activity. The conclusion was that physically active older adults are, indeed, more socially connected. The Netz et al. study (Netz, Goldsmith et al., 2012) focused on feeling lonely as related to physical activity. The findings showed that feelings of loneliness, but not living alone, were associated with lower odds of engaging in physical activity.

Interestingly, both studies reported a seemingly dose-dependent relationship between physical activity and social connectedness. The dose in the Netz et al. study (2012) was measured by the level of physical activity, while in the Litwin study (2003) the dose was attributed to the diversity of social connectedness. In the Netz et al. study (2012) the rate of reporting loneliness was highest in the inactive group, followed by the insufficiently active group, and was lowest in the sufficiently active group. Importantly, this dose-dependent relationship was indicated in all the study groups: men, women, Jews, Arabs, religious people, and secular people. In the Litwin study (2003) the highest percentage of people reporting being physically active was indicated by the most extended social network—the diverse, followed by the friends-network which is the second diverse-network, followed by the neighbor-network which is more limited in terms of social ties, followed by the family-network and the restricted-network, in which people reported the least social ties.

It should be noted that the association between social connectedness and physical activity in both studies assumed that the social component affects one's likelihood of engaging in physical activity. The opposite direction is also possible. That is, older adults who are physically active might maintain more diverse social ties, or feel less lonely as a result of their improved physical state. In sum, physically active adults are more socially connected. And feelings of loneliness, but not living alone, are associated with lower odds of engaging in physical activity. Last, there is a dose-dependent (negative) relationship between rate of reporting loneliness and physical activity in all population groups: men, women, Jews, Arabs, religious, and secular people. As the diversity of social connections becomes higher, there is greater likelihood of engaging in physical activity.

Physical activity and psychological function

In the *Mabat Zahav Survey*, physical activity was also investigated in relation to psychological functioning. Two psychological components were examined: mental health and cognitive functioning (Netz, Dunsky et al., 2012):

Mental health: As positive and negative aspects of mental health measure different facets of psychological distress, this study explored the positive and negative aspects of mental health separately, assessed by good and bad feelings, respectively, in relation to physical activity. Results indicated that adherence to the recommended guidelines of physical activity in older adults in Israel is a small but significant contributor to the explanation of psychological functioning in addition to, and independent of, demographic and health variables. In both aspects of mental health—the positive as well as the negative, the sufficiently active—those who met the recommended guideline of physical activity—were superior to both the insufficiently active and inactive groups. However, only in the negative factor was a dose-dependent relationship observed, with the fewest bad feelings in the sufficiently active individuals, more in the insufficiently active, and the most in the inactive group.

Cognitive functioning: A clear dose-dependent relationship was indicated between adherence to the recommended dose of physical activity and the likelihood of cognitive impairment. However, after controlling for demographic and health variables, the additional contribution of physical activity to account for cognitive functioning was quite small. Adherence to the recommended guidelines of physical activity is a small but significant contributor to the explanation of psychological functioning in addition to, and independent of, demographic and health variables. There is also a dose-dependent relationship between negative effects (bad feelings) and level of physical activity, with those who meet official guidelines of physical activity having fewer bad feelings. Furthermore, there is a dose-dependent relationship between adherence to physical activity guidelines and the likelihood of cognitive impairment.

Physical activity, function, and longevity

The Jerusalem longitudinal study focusing on 70+ old people is probably the most comprehensive study on health, functioning, health behavior, and mortality in older adults in Israel, devoting a great deal of investigation to the benefits of physical activity to health and longevity (Jacobs et al., 2013; Stessman et al. 2009; Stessman & Jacobs, 2014). This study followed an age-homogeneous cohort of Jerusalem residents who were 70 years old in 1990, in three phases: at age 70, at age 78, and at age 85. Participants were asked about the frequency of physical activity in which they were engaged. The answers were: (1) less than 4 hours weekly, (2) about 4 hours weekly, (3) vigorous sports at least twice weekly (e.g., jogging or swimming), and (4) regular physical activity (e.g., walking at least an hour daily). Physical activity was dichotomized as sedentary (answer to 1) vs. physically active (answers to 2, 3, and 4).

Physical activity and longevity: Two publications focused on physical activity and longevity, with one reporting the results after the second phase (Stessman et al., 2000) and the other after the third phase (Stessman et al., 2009). Based on the dichotomized distinction between sedentary and active participants, the findings indicated that continuing—but more importantly also initiating—physical activity among older people delays functional deterioration and improves survival. A unique and unprecedented finding was that the magnitude of the difference between physically active and sedentary participants actually increased with advancing age, with the maximum survival benefits observed among the oldest age group. On the other hand, an analysis of survival according to the four physical activity levels found no clear dose-dependent effect.

Physical activity and longevity in Diabetes Mellitus: Remarkably, the authors observed the same results in a subgroup of the sample—participants with Type 2 Diabetes Mellitus (Stessman & Jacobs, 2014). Physical activity was associated with improved survival in this group, and this benefit of physical activity continued in the oldest old group. Furthermore, the magnitude of benefit observed in this subgroup was comparable to, and even greater than the survival benefit associated with physical activity among similar aged non-diabetic older people.

Holocaust survivors in the Jerusalem Study: Another subgroup of the sample were Holocaust survivors who were assessed 50 years following the Holocaust, at age 70 and 77, on various health and health behavior characteristics (Stessman et al., 2008). In terms of physical activity, they reported engaging in less physical activity than the controls. However, while results showed that they had impaired functional status and social characteristics, in measures of physical health, patterns of decline, and overall mortality they were comparable to the rest of the study population.

Physical activity and health service utilization: An interesting and under-studied issue that was investigated in the Jerusalem study is the impact of changing physical activity levels on health service use among the oldest old age group (Jacobs et al., 2013). This issue is critical in light of the tremendous demand for medical services in older adults, reflecting population growth as well as the rise of comorbidity, loss of independence, and increasing medical needs in this group. Findings indicated that not only continuing to be physically active, but also initiating physical activity at a very advanced age, is associated with reduced emergency room visits and hospitalization.

Conclusion

While Israel is a relatively young country, life expectancy in Israel is one of the highest in the world. This means that not only is the number of older adults in Israel relatively high, but also the percentage of the very old, aged 80+, is dramatically increasing. Furthermore, so far a large percentage of Jewish older adults—especially in the very old—are not Israeli-born. Their perception on physical activity may be influenced by their country of origin, which may not always value the benefits of a physically active lifestyle in promoting mental and physical health, and in preventing chronic diseases and functional deterioration.

Consequently, a large section of older adults in Israel—both Jews and Arabs—still relate to the "well-earned rest" myth that provides the "legitimacy" to conducting sedentary life. This adds to another myth, still prevalent in those of advanced age, that if you are chronically ill you are not allowed to exercise. An interesting excuse sometimes used in the past by Jewish older adults for not exercising, is the perception of the Jewish people as "the people of the Book"—meaning that physical activity is a waste of time. This trend, however, is changing. While previous data indicated that about one-third of older adults meet the official WHO guidelines of physical activity, in the most recent data there is an increase in people meeting the official guidelines. This increase, however, is not shown in the Arab older adults. In the most recent data available, there is a large gap between Jews and Arabs, with over 40 percent of Jews meeting the guidelines and only about 19 percent among Arab men and 6 percent in Arab women. Interestingly, among Jews the rate of meeting the guidelines in men is over 40 percent in all age groups, and in women the rate of meeting the guidelines is higher in age 65+ than in all age groups. In the Arab population, this trend is reversed: as age increases, the rate of physical activity decreases, especially among women.

In addition to using data drawn from governmental publications, this chapter reviewed all scientific publications on physical activity and health in advanced age, based on a large random sample of older adult Israelis. While most publications reviewed in this chapter were published in 2009–2016, the data analyzed in these studies were gathered 5 to 7 years prior to the publication year. This means that the information described in this chapter may not be the most updated. On the other hand, there are a few trends that are consistent and are repeated in most studies—some of them 10 years apart, for example the increase in physical activity in successive samples. Furthermore, these trends are also typical to most OECD countries, which are similar to Israel in quite a few demographic aspects—such as life expectancy, health, education, etc. In addition, although physical activity was measured differently in the various publications, the trends of the relationship between physical activity and health are similar in all of them. In older adults in Israel, more men than women, more Jews than Arabs, and more secular than religious people (in both Hews and Arabs) adhere to physical activity guidelines recommended by official organizations; and walking is the most frequently reported physical activity. Based on longitudinal studies of the same cohort, as people get older they are less active; however, based on successive cohorts, there is an increase in physical activity in old age. There is clearly a positive relationship, in most cases dose-dependent, between physical activity and the following components: health, longevity, social connectedness, emotional and cognitive functioning.

References

American College of Sports Medicine (ACSM). (2009). Exercise and physical activity for older adults. *Medicine & Science in Sports & Exercise, 41*(7), 1510–1530.

Cohen-Mansfield, J. (2012). Trends in health behaviours in the old-old population: results from a National Survey. *Behavioural Medicine, 38*(1), 6–11.

Cohen-Mansfield, J. & Kivity, Y. (2011). The relationships among health behaviours in older persons. *Journal of Aging and Health, 23*(5), 822–842.

Cohen-Mansfield, J., Shmotkin, D., & Goldberg, S. (2010). Predictors of longitudinal changes in older adults' physical activity engagement. *Journal of Aging and Physical Activity, 18*(2), 141–157.

Dunsky, A. Zach, S., Zeev, A., Goldbourt, U., Shimony, T., Goldsmith, R., & Netz, Y. (2014). Level of physical activity and anthropometric characteristics in old age – results from a national health survey. *European Review of Aging and Physical Activity, 11*(2), 149. DOI 10.1007/s11556-014-0139-y.

Israel Aging Population (2017). http://medicine.jrank.org/pages/938/Israel-Aging-population.html.

Jacobs, J. M., Rottenberg, Y., Cohen, A., & Stessman, J. (2013). Physical activity and health service utilization among older people. *Journal of the American Medical Directors Association, 14*(2), 125–129.

Jewish Virtual Library (2017). www.jewishvirtuallibrary.org/latest-population-statistics-for-israelodox.

Litwin, H. (2003). Social predictors of physical activity in later life: the contribution of social-network type. *Journal of Aging and Physical Activity, 11*(3), 389–406.

MASHAV Planning for the Elderly—A National Data Base Israel: Israel's Elderly—Facts and Figures 2015. http://brookdale.jdc.org.il/_Uploads/dbsAttachedFiles/Israel-s-Elderly-Facts-and-Figures-2015.pdf.

Ministry of Health, Israel, Centre for Disease Control (ICDC), Publication 371, Highlights of Health in Israel, 2016. www.health.gov.il/publicationsfiles/highlights_of_health_in_israel2016.pdf.

Netz, Y., Dunsky, A., Zach, S., Goldsmith, R., T. Shimony, T., Goldbourt, U., & Zeev, A. (2012). Psychological functioning and adherence to the recommended dose of physical activity in later life: results from a national health survey. *International Psychogeriatrics, 24*(12), 2027–2036.

Netz, Y., Goldsmith, R., Shimony, T., Ben-Moshe, Y., & Zeev, A. (2011). Adherence to physical activity recommendations in older adults – results from the "Mabat Zahav" Israel National Health and Nutrition Survey. *Journal of Aging and Physical Activity, 19*(1), 30–47.

Netz, Y., Goldsmith, R., Shimony, T., Arnon, M., & Zeev, A. (2012). Loneliness is associated with an increased risk of sedentary life in older Israelis. *Aging & Mental Health, 17*(1), 40–47. DOI:10.1080/13607863.2012.715140.

Stessman, J. & Jacobs, J. M. (2014). Diabetes mellitus, physical activity, and longevity between the ages of 70 and 90. *Journal of the American Geriatric Society, 62*(7), 1329–1334.

Stessman, J., Cohen, A., Hammerman-Rozenberg, R., Bursztyn, M., Azoulay, D., Maaravi, Y., & Jacobs, J. (2008). Holocaust survivors in old age: the Jerusalem Longitudinal Study. *Journal of the American Geriatric Society, 56*, 470–477.

Stessman, J., Hammerman-Rozenberg, R., Cohen, A., Ein-Mor, E., & Jacobs, J. M. (2009). Physical activity, function, and longevity among the very old. *Archives of Internal Medicine, 169*(16), 1476–1483.

Stessman, J., Maaravi, R., Hammerman-Rozenberg, R., & Cohen, A. (2000). The effects of physical activity on mortality in the Jerusalem 70-year-olds Longitudinal Study. *Journal of the American Geriatric Society, 48*(5), 499–504.

Chapter 11

Aging, health, and physical activity in Iran

Maryam Koushkie Jahromi

Introduction

The world is aging in several parts of the globe, and Iran is no exception. This chapter presents an analysis of the well-being and physical activity of older adults in Iran. In 2000, the percentage of older adults (aged over 60 years) around the world was 10 percent, and in 2050, it is anticipated to be 22 percent. In 2000, the proportion of older adults was significantly higher (20 percent) in more developed countries compared to the less developed countries where it was closer to 8 percent. This disparity is expected to continue in 2050, from 33 percent in developed countries to 21 percent in less developed countries (Mirkin & Weinberger, 2001).

Aging in Iran

Iran was known as Persia before 1935. The Islamic Republic of Iran is located in the Eastern Mediterranean region, and it is the eighteenth largest country in the world in terms of area at 1,648,195 km and the fourth largest country in Asia. According to the 2016 census, the population of Iran is about 80 million (51 percent male and 49 percent female). The country is diverse in origin, reflecting distinct waves of migration into the country, as well as its conquest by numerous powers throughout history. The official religion is Shiite Islam, practiced by about 90 percent of the population and most of the remainder are Sunni Muslims with about 2 percent non-Muslim religious minorities, including Bahá'ís, Mandeans, Hindus, Sikhs, Yezidis, Yarsanis, Zoroastrians, Jews, and Christians (Central Intelligence Agency, 2015).

Increased life expectancy has resulted in an increase in the percentage of older adults in Iran. However, there are significant differences in life expectancy based on cultural and economic factors, as well as political conflict such as the 8-year Iran-Iraq war. The life expectancy of Iranians has been estimated as 74.6 years for women and 72.1 years for men in 2012 (Islamic Republic News Agency, 2012; Statistical Centre of Iran,

2017). In Iran, the older adult population is also expected to increase from 9 percent to 10 percent in 2021, and 21 percent (about 26 million) by 2050 (Islamic Republic News Agency, 2012).

Census data indicate that among older adults in Iran during two consecutive census studies that those aged 30 to 64 make up 39.3 percent in 2011 and 44.8 percent in 2016; while those aged 65 and over make up 5.7 percent and 6.1 percent respectively. The ratio of the older adults in the rural areas is higher than in urban areas, although the life expectancy in rural areas is somewhat lower than the urban areas (Statistical Centre of Iran, 2017). The main reason for the higher proportion of elders in rural areas may be due to the migration of the rural population, especially younger adults to urban areas. Retirement age is 45 for disabled adults and 50 for others in Iran. Such a young retirement age (Sohofi Parast, 2008) may be used as an incentive for retirement to provide more jobs for younger adults for whom unemployment is high (Statistics, 2012). Although some older men and women do seek other forms of employment and/or begin businesses after retirement.

There are significant gendered differences in the occupations of older men and women. Women comprise a lower percentage of the work force and tend to retire, on average, 5 years earlier than men (Kiani & Bayanzadeh, 2010). As a result, older women also tend to face more economic challenges than older men. A limited number of older adults (0.24 percent) live in formal elder care centers. Cultural traditions and religious beliefs dictate that taking care of aging parents is a moral virtue (Tajvar, Arab, & Montazeri, 2008). As a result, it is generally family members who care for elders, although a variety of factors can influence family care quality including socioeconomic class, education, health care knowledge and skills, cultural movements, and health status of the old persons (Hedayati, Hadi, Mostafavi, Akbarzadeh, & Montazeri, 2014).

Aging is generally accompanied by physiological, health, and psychological changes. Numerous studies have found that physical activity can moderate such changes. Engagement in physical activity is dependent on a number of inter-related cultural, environmental, and socioeconomic situations. Health is perhaps the major factor impacting activity. Additionally, many social and cultural buffers and barriers can either promote or hinder participation in physical activity. The remainder of this chapter addresses these factors as they pertain to physical activity and aging in Iran.

Aging and health status

Older adults tend to suffer from more chronic diseases, physical disabilities, mental illnesses, and other co-morbidities (Boutayeb & Boutayeb, 2005). Determinants of health include social concerns (e.g., being supported by family), treatment (Sethi et al., 2011), information about aging and risk factors (Song et al., 2013), nutritional status (Borden, Conner, & MPA-HAS, 2012), psycho-emotional concerns (mental stress, emotional support (World Health Organization, 2003)), financial circumstances (Song et al., 2013), availability of health care (Borden, Conner, & MPA-HAS, 2012; Song et al., 2013), and physical status (Borden, Conner, & MPA-HAS, 2012). Common concerns in Iran include malnutrition, falls, and cognitive dysfunction. Generally, men and women suffer from the similar health problems, but the frequency and outcomes of these problems differ.

Support and well-being

According to some studies, religious participation is directly and positively related to mental and physical health (Lawler-Row & Elliott, 2009). The role of religion has been confirmed in the well-being of older adults. Living with family generally enhances health among older adults. A lack of social support, by contrast, has been shown to increase the risk for mortality (Dhar, 2001). Studies indicate that some determinants of ill health are primarily behavioral risk factors related to lifestyle. These include tobacco use, poor diet, physical inactivity, and alcohol misuse which all account for over one-third of global chronic diseases (Scarborough et al., 2011).

Gerontologists have focused on ways of increasing both the quality and the quantity of life (Drewnowsk et al., 2003). Clearly the major solution to such a concern is the development of social policies that promote healthy aging (United Kingdom Department of Health, 2004). Healthy aging is a lifelong process based on contextual as well as physical, social, and mental factors (Health Canada, 2004).

The United Nations research agenda on aging for the 21st century (United Nations Office on Ageing, 2003) expressed the need for research on the determinants of healthy aging as a priority so that the effective preventive, curative, and rehabilitative methods of intervention can be applied (Peel, McClure, & Bartlett, 2005). Body composition, functional fitness, psycho-social factors, and the prevention of falls have been considered as important correlations to positive health and are related to the quality of life in later adulthood (Gouveia et al., 2017). These factors are influenced by exercise and activity.

Later life and well-being in Iran

Older men's and women's abilities to engage in physical activity is influenced by a number of factors. For example, studies indicate that the quality of life in later adulthood is significantly impacted by a variety of mental health concerns, the most prominent one being depression. Additional concerns include financial deficiencies and limitations associated with chronic illness. Positive and satisfying relationships improve well-being and promote activity (Netuveli, Wiggins, Hildon, Montgomery, & Blane, 2006). Borowiak and Kostka (2004) found a decreased quality of life in elders taken care of at home compared to institutions and found that physical and cognitive function deficits, overweight/obesity, and lack of regular physical activity are the most important predictors of decreased quality of life in home-dwelling elders.

Aging is clearly accompanied by a decrease in the quality of life. It is, however, important to note that cultural differences may exist in this decrease. Molzahn, Kalfoss, Makaroff, and Skevington (2011) evaluated quality of life in 22 countries and found considerable differences in various aspects relating to quality of life for people living in medium and high-development countries. Culture appeared to account for 15.9 percent of the variance in the priority ratings of quality of life. Cultural differences were reduced once health status, gender, and age were taken into account.

Clearly the quality of the aging experience varies by culture. A study by Nasirzadeh et al. (2014) found that older adults had differing responses to questions assessing the quality of their life and income: 95 percent stated it was moderate, 4.5 percent unfavorable, and 0.5 percent favorable. Moderate-income elder women and educated elders had a better lifestyle and recommended education of healthy lifestyle. A meta-analysis research conducted by Cheraghi, Doosti-Irani, Nedjat, Cheraghi, and Nedjat (2017) indicated that the mean score of the quality of life in the elderly population of Iran was less than the mean score of the quality of life (76.95) in the general population of Iran (Koohi, Nedjat, Yaseri, & Cheraghi, 2016). According to this study, all mean scores of quality of life were less than the reported scores of the study by Skevington, Lotfy, and O'Connell (2004) (obtained from information from 23 countries), including: physical health (54.6 vs. 63.7), psychological health (57.3 vs. 63.1), social relationship (57.9 vs. 63.7), and environmental health (51.6 vs. 61.2). Comparing quality of life in men and women indicated that quality of life in men is better than women, which may be due to higher socioeconomic status, having supportive families, having more satisfying social support in society, having a higher level of education, and better job position among Iranian elders. The authors concluded that although the findings of the study were limited to three provinces in Iran and because of the heterogeneity of Iranian culture and other effective factors, the overall findings of the entire may differ.

Another meta-analysis review by Farajzadeh, Gheshlagh, and Sayehmiri (2017) concluded that the quality of life among the Iranian elders, according to about 21 articles, was almost at an "average" level, and the year of study or region was not effective on findings. Quality of life was lower in sick (especially fibromyalgia and rheumatoid arthritis patients) elders than healthy people, which confirms the priority of health status to culture stated by Molzahn, Kalfoss, Makaroff, and Skevington (2011).

Economical, sociocultural, educational, and health care circumstances may have an effect on the quality of life of elderly people (Farzianpour, Hosseini, Rostami, Pordanjani, & Hosseini, 2012). Based on the statistics, approximately 20 percent of adults older than 70 and 50 percent of adults older than 85 are dependent on others for daily activities (Hellström, Persson, & Hallberg, 2004). A study in Iran found that one in four older adults suffered from severe disabilities (Adib-Hajbaghery, 2011). The most prevalent causes of disability in Iranian adults in 2010 were heart disease (22.77 percent), neoplasms (9.48 percent), and lower back pain (5.72 percent) (Namazi et al., 2015). The primary causes of death and morbidity in Iran for those over the age of 50 was related to dietary risks, high blood pressure, high body mass index, physical inactivity, smoking, and ambient particulate matter pollution (Forouzanfar et al., 2014).

Physical activity in later life

Older adults often struggle with limitations of personal abilities in daily activity, which cause dependence on others. An active life style can delay aging and prevent functional decline, especially activity abilities, and improve health and quality of life (Brandon, Boyette, Gaasch, & Lloyd, 2000; Singh, 2002; Walker, 2002; Hillsdon, Brunner, Guralnik, & Marmot, 2005). Physical activity is the most effective way to prevent and control many non-communicable diseases (Malina & Little, 2008). The World Health Organization has introduced physical activity as one of the important components of health, especially in later life (de Souza Vale, de Oliveira, Pernambuco, da Silva Novaes, & de Andrade, 2009). It is estimated that low physical activity causes 1.9 million deaths and 19 million disabilities every year throughout the world. For instance, studies have indicated that low physical activity is the cause of 10 percent–16 percent of diabetes and a sedentary lifestyle is closely related to breast, colon, and rectal cancers (WHO, 2002).

Physical activity in later life provides personal independence, physical strength, and quality of life, and plays a role in the prevention of specific diseases such as dementia and Alzheimer's (Logan, Gottlieb, Maitland, Meegan, & Spriet, 2013). It is also effective in preventing and treating high blood pressure, cardiovascular diseases, arthritis, and osteoporosis (Struber, 2004). Physical activity is directly correlated with reducing depression and anxiety among older adults (Cooney, Dwan, & Mead, 2014). Physical activity can reduce the risk of cerebral diseases and complications related to aging (Ivey, Hafer-Macko, & Macko, 2006). Many findings have proved the positive effect of physical activity on reducing or controlling obesity, improving muscle strength, reducing other cardiovascular risk factors such as low density lipoprotein (LDL), cholesterol, and triglyceride in elders (de Souza Vale, de Oliveira, Pernambuco, da Silva Novaes, & de Andrade, 2009).

Physical activity can result in active aging by improving psychological health, preventing and managing chronic diseases, premature death, illness, and disability, which leads to improving quality of life as well as independence (Seniors BC, 2012). Regular and adequate physical activity has been demonstrated to improve functional ability through enhancing physiological aspects, such as maximal aerobic capacity (Vincent, Braith, Feldman, Kallas, & Lowenthal, 2002), muscle strength, coordination, and balance function (Barnett, Smith, Lord, Williams, & Baumand, 2003), and walking speed (Lopopolo, Greco, Sullivan, Craik, & Mangione, 2006) which can help older people remain independent for the longest period of time (Spirduso & Cronin, 2001). Active living improves social relationships through positive mental effects and exercise/activity situations. Therefore, older adults who engage in regular physical activity can also experience economic advantages by increasing their independency and reducing medical costs. Achieving optimal age is associated with being active.

Despite all these benefits, high proportions of elders in most countries lead sedentary lives (Schutzer & Graves, 2004). These are a number of inter-related determinants of active aging including economic factors, availability of health and social services, social, personal, and behavioral determinants.

Physical activity across the life span

An individual's physical activity level in later life is related to the level of activity they are accustomed to throughout their lives. Activity across the life span tends to continue into later life. As mentioned previously, physical activity is generally influenced by such factors as socioeconomic and cultural values and norms, as well as environmental and social circumstances (Watt, Carson, Lawlor, Patel, & Ebrahim, 2009). However, activity level tends to decline in later life. Studies have indicated that sedentary behavior is more common in later life than earlier in life (Baloh, Ying, & Jacobson, 2003). This is unfortunate, as a reduction of physical activity in aging tends to accelerate aging related declines in health (Benjamin & Donnelly, 2013).

Physical activity patterns vary by country and region. For example, in Brazil only 13.7 percent of elders were physically active and 80.7 percent had low physical activity or were not active at all (Dias-da-Costa et al., 2005). In England, only 10 percent of men and 2 percent of women aged about 75 years and older were found to be active (Mavritsakis & Ghidrai, 2009); regardless, these percentages tend to be low. Iranian elders also vary in their activity levels. Activity levels for Iranian elders tend to be based on many related factors. Researchers in 2006 in Yazd (the central city of Iran) found that the physical activity level in urban populations was low and 68.4 percent of the population over 60 years was, in fact, physically inactive (Motefaker et al., 2007). Another study in Isfahan (central city of Iran) indicated that only 13.7 percent of the elders had adequate physical activity (Eshaghi, Shahsanai, & Ardakani, 2011).

A study of activity levels among older adults in Kashan (central city of Iran) indicated that out of 400 older aged (over 60 years) participants, 320 and 59 people had low and moderate physical activity levels, respectively, and only one of the participants engaged in regular high levels of physical activity. Men were more likely to be moderately or extremely physically active. A significant relationship was found between physical activity and gender, marital status, educational status, current occupation, and personal independence. This study found that, in general, there were low levels of physical activity among older adults in Kashan (Sadrollahi, Hosseinian, Alavi, Khalili, & Esalatmanesh, 2016). A review study of physical activity in all age groups of Iran indicated that most of the studies reported high prevalence of physical inactivity (Fakhrzadeh et al., 2016).

There are barriers and facilitators for physical activity among older adults. Some factors, including social, recreational, environmental, demographic, and psychological factors, are related to physical activity during older age (Trost, Owen, Bauman, Sallis, & Brown, 2002). It is obvious that activity barriers are different among people (Koohsari, Karakiewicz, & Kaczynski; Trost, Owen, Bauman, Sallis, & Brown, 2002). The report of Centers for Disease Control and Prevention in 2007 showed that 14 percent of elder people aged 65 through 74 years and 7 percent of elders over the age of 75 had regular physical activity (Anderson-Hanley, Snyder, Nimon, & Arciero, 2011). Rimmer, Wang, and Smith (2008) reported that elders suffering from cerebral stroke and barriers to physical activity were the result of lack of information about physical activity centers and lack of fitness and motivation. Siddiqi, Tiro, and Shuval (2011) found that shortage of time, physical health problems, and probable injuries are important barriers to physical activity for elders.

Researchers in Tehran (Iran) indicated that the most important barrier of physical activity for elders was a lack of motivation (Salehi, Taghdisi, Ghasemi, & Shokervash, 2010). Mosallanezhad, Hörder, Salavati, Nilsson-Wikmar, and Frändin (2012) evaluated and compared the physical activity of Iranian elders and found that 75-year-old Iranians were less physically active than their Swedish peers and their functional performance was worse. Similar gender differences were also identified, with women being less active than men. Iranians who took a daily walk of at least 30 minutes indicated positive effects on most health-related aspects and functional performance.

Conclusion

Research conducted on physical activity among older Iranian adults found that the quality of life and physical activity of older Iranians is not adequate. This lack of physical activity among older adults may be related to inactivity habits in previous ages of childhood or young adulthood or the Iranian culture to take care of elders with family, but not having enough information or plans about their health necessities, especially their physical activity. Some other barriers of physical activity in the older adult population may be due to a lack of available facilities such as parks, gyms, and walking trails. In conclusion, while engaging in regular physical activity is a vital component of maintaining health and well-being in later life, there are certain steps that need to be taken in order to help older adults become and stay active. These steps include the development of programs that can provide support, the development of safe walking spaces, and education on the importance of physical activity as well as related health care information.

References

Adib-Hajbaghery, M. (2011). Evaluation of old-age disability and related factors among an Iranian elderly population/Evaluation de l'incapacite liee a l'age et des facteurs y afferents dans une population de personnes agees en Iran. *Eastern Mediterranean Health Journal*, *17*(9), 671.

Anderson-Hanley, C., Snyder, A. L., Nimon, J. P., & Arciero, P. J. (2011). Social facilitation in virtual reality-enhanced exercise: competitiveness moderates exercise effort of older adults. *Clinical Intervention & Aging*, *6*, 275–280.

Baloh, R. W., Ying, S. H., & Jacobson, K. M. (2003). A longitudinal study of gait and balance dysfunction in normal older people. *Archives of Neurology*, *60*(6), 835–839.

Barnett, A., Smith, B., Lord, S. R., Williams, M., & Baumand, A. (2003). Community-based group exercise improves balance and reduces falls in at-risk older people: a randomised controlled trial. *Age and Ageing*, *32*(4), 407–414.

Benjamin, K. & Donnelly, T. T. (2013). Barriers and facilitators influencing the physical activity of Arabic adults: a literature review. *Avicenna*, *8*, 2–16.

Borden, C., Conner, C., & MPA-HAS, B. S. N. (2012). Nutrition for older adults. In L. Hark, K. Ashton, & D. Deen (Eds.) *The Nurse Practitioner's Guide to Nutrition* (pp. 113–133). Ames, IO: Wiley-Blackwell.

Borowiak, E. & Kostka, T. (2004). Predictors of quality of life in older people living at home and in institutions. *Aging Clinical and Experimental Research*, *16*(3), 212–220.

Boutayeb, A. & Boutayeb, S. (2005). The burden of non-communicable diseases in developing countries. *International Journal for Equity in Health*, *4*(1), 2.

Brandon, L. J., Boyette, L. W., Gaasch, D. A., & Lloyd, A. (2000). Effects of lower extremity strength training on functional mobility in older adults. *Journal of Aging and Physical Activity*, *8*(3), 214–227.

Central Intelligence Agency (Ed.). (2015). Iran people 2015, *The world fact book 2014–15*. Retrieved from: https://photius.com/world_fact_book_2015/iran/iran_people.html.

Cheraghi, Z., Doosti-Irani, A., Nedjat, S., Cheraghi, P., & Nedjat, S. (2016). Quality of life in elderly Iranian population using the QOL-brief questionnaire: a systematic review. *Iranian Journal of Public Health, 45*(8), 978.

Cooney, G., Dwan, K., & Mead, G. (2014). Exercise for depression. *JAMA, 311*(23), 2432–2433.

De Souza Vale, R. G., de Oliveira, R. D., Pernambuco, C. S., da Silva Novaes, J., & de Andrade, A. D. F. D. (2009). Effects of muscle strength and aerobic training on basal serum levels of IGF-1 and cortisol in elderly women. *Archives of Gerontology and Geriatrics, 49*(3), 343–347.

Dhar, H. L. (2001). Gender, aging, health and society. *The Journal of the Association of Physicians of India, 49*, 1012–1020.

Dias-da-Costa, J. S., Hallal, P. C., Wells, J. C. K., Daltoé, T., Fuchs, S. C., Menezes, A. M. B., & Olinto, M. T. A. (2005). Epidemiology of leisure-time physical activity: a population-based study in southern Brazil. *Cadernos de Saúde Pública, 21*(1), 275–282.

Drewnowski, A., Monsen, E., Birkett, D., Gunther, S., Vendeland, S., Su, J., & Marshall, G. (2003). Health screening and health promotion programmes for the elderly. *Disease Management & Health Outcomes, 11*(5), 299–309.

Eshaghi, S. R., Shahsanai, A., & Ardakani, M. M. (2011). Assessment of the physical activity of elderly population of Isfahan, Iran. *Journal of Isfahan Medical School, 29*(147), 939–956.

Fakhrzadeh, H., Djalalinia, S., Mirarefin, M., Arefirad, T., Asayesh, H., Safiri, S., Samami, E., Mansourian, M., Shamsizadeh, M., & Qorbani, M. (2016). Prevalence of physical inactivity in Iran: a systematic review. *Journal of Cardiovascular and Thoracic Research, 8*(3), 92–97.

Farajzadeh, M., Gheshlagh, R. G., & Sayehmiri, K. (2017). Health related quality of life in Iranian elderly citizens: a systematic review and meta-analysis. *International Journal of Community Based Nursing and Midwifery, 5*(2), 100–111.

Farzianpour, F., Hosseini, S., Rostami, M., Pordanjani, S. B., & Hosseini, S. M. (2012). Quality of life of the elderly residents. *American Journal of Applied Sciences, 9*(1), 71.

Forouzanfar, M. H., Sepanlou, S. G., Shahraz, S., Dicker, D., Naghavi, P., Pourmalek, F., Mokdad, A., Lozano, R., Vos, T., Asadi-Lari, M., Sayyari, A.A., Murray, C., & Naghavi, M. (2014). Evaluating causes of death and morbidity in Iran, global burden of diseases, injuries, and risk factors study 2010. *Archives of Iranian Medicine, 17*(5), 304.

Gouveia, É. R. Q., Gouveia, B. R., Ihle, A., Kliegel, M., Maia, J. A., i Badia, S. B., & Freitas, D. L. (2017). Correlates of health-related quality of life in young-old and old–old community-dwelling older adults. *Quality of Life Research, 26*(6), 1561–1569.

Health Canada. (2004). Workshop on healthy aging. Retrieved from: www.hc-sc.gc.ca/ seniors-sines/pubs/workshop_healthyaging/pdf/workshop1_e.pdf. Accessed February 10, 2004.

Hedayati, H. R., Hadi, N., Mostafavi, L., Akbarzadeh, A., & Montazeri, A. (2014). Quality of life among nursing home residents compared with the elderly at home. *Shiraz E-Medical Journal, 15*(4), e22718.

Hellström, Y., Persson, G., & Hallberg, I. R. (2004). Quality of life and symptoms among older people living at home. *Journal of Advanced Nursing, 48*(6), 584–593.

Hillsdon, M. M., Brunner, E. J., Guralnik, J. M., & Marmot, M. G. (2005). Prospective study of physical activity and physical function in early old age. *American Journal of Preventive Medicine, 28*(3), 245–250.

Islamic Republic News Agency (IRNA). Life expectancy has increased in Iran. Retrieved from: www.irna.com/News/80254515.

Ivey, F. M., Hafer-Macko, C. E., & Macko, R. F. (2006). Exercise rehabilitation after stroke. *NeuroRx, 3*(4), 439–450.

Kiani, S. & Bayanzadeh, M. (2010). The Iranian population is graying: are we ready? *Archives of Iranian Medicine, 13*(4), 333.

Koohi, F., Nedjat, S., Yaseri, M., & Cheraghi, Z. (2017). Quality of life among general populations of different countries in the past 10 years, with a focus on Human Development Index: a systematic review and meta-analysis. *Iranian Journal of Public Health, 46*(1), 12–22.

Koohsari, M. J., Karakiewicz, J. A., & Kaczynski, A. T. (2013). Public open space and walking: the role of proximity, perceptual qualities of the surrounding built environment, and street configuration. *Environment and Behaviour, 45*(6), 706–736.

Lawler-Row, K. A. & Elliott, J. (2009). The role of religious activity and spirituality in the health and well-being of older adults. *Journal of Health Psychology, 14*(1), 43–52.

Logan, S. L., Gottlieb, B. H., Maitland, S. B., Meegan, D., & Spriet, L. L. (2013). The Physical Activity Scale for the Elderly (PASE) questionnaire; does it predict physical health? *International Journal of Environmental Research and Public Health, 10*(9), 3967–3986.

Lopopolo, R. B., Greco, M., Sullivan, D., Craik, R. L., & Mangione, K. K. (2006). Effect of therapeutic exercise on gait speed in community-dwelling elderly people: a meta-analysis. *Physical Therapy, 86*(4), 520.

Malina, R. M. & Little, B. B. (2008). Physical activity: the present in the context of the past. *American Journal of Human Biology, 20*(4), 373–391.

Mavritsakis, N. & Ghidrai, O. (2009). Activitatea fizică şi iatrogeniile psihice la vârstnici. *Palestrica of the Third Millennium Civilization & Sport, 10*(3), 298–302.

Mirkin, B. & Weinberger, M. B. (2001). The demography of population ageing. *Publicado en Population Bulletin of the United Nations, 42*(43), 37–53.

Molzahn, A. E., Kalfoss, M., Makaroff, K. S., & Skevington, S. M. (2011). Comparing the importance of different aspects of quality of life to older adults across diverse cultures. *Age and Ageing, 40*(2), 192–199.

Mosallanezhad, Z., Hörder, H., Salavati, M., Nilsson-Wikmar, L., & Frändin, K. (2012). Physical activity and physical functioning in Swedish and Iranian 75-year-olds – a comparison. *Archives of Gerontology and Geriatrics, 55*(2), 422–430.

Motefaker, M., Sadrbafghi, S. M., Rafiee, M., Bahadorzadeh, L., Namayandeh, S. M., Karimi, M., & Abdoli, A. M. (2007). Epidemiology of physical activity: a population based study in Yazd cityide attempt and its relation to stressors and supportive systems: a study in Karaj city. *Tehran University Medical Journal TUMS Publications*, 65(4), 77–81.

Namazi, S., Saeedi, M., Sharifi, F., Fadayevatan, R., Nabavizadeh, F., Delavari, A., & Naderimagham, S. H. (2015). The most prevalent causes of deaths, DALYs, and geriatric syndromes in Iranian elderly people between 1990 and 2010: findings from the global burden of disease study 2010. *Archives of Iranian Medicine*, 18(8), 462–479.

Nasirzadeh, M., Gholami, L., Jalilian, F., Aligol, M., Bakhtiari, M. H., Mahboubi, M., & Matin, B. K. (2014). Status of lifestyle in Iranian elderly population. *Journal of Science and Today*, 1(3), 114–116.

Netuveli, G., Wiggins, R. D., Hildon, Z., Montgomery, S. M., & Blane, D. (2006). Quality of life at older ages: evidence from the English longitudinal study of aging (wave 1). *Journal of Epidemiology and Community Health*, 60(4), 357–363.

Peel, N. M., McClure, R. J., & Bartlett, H. P. (2005). Behavioural determinants of healthy aging. *American Journal of Preventive Medicine*, 28(3), 298–304.

People, H. & US Department of Health and Human Services. (2010). Healthy people 2010. *Services USDoAaUSDoHaH, editor*. Washington, DC.

Rimmer, J. H., Wang, E., & Smith, D. (2008). Barriers associated with exercise and community access for individuals with stroke. *Journal of Rehabilitation Research and Development*, 45(2), 315.

Sadrollahi, A., Hosseinian, M., Alavi, N. M., Khalili, Z., & Esalatmanesh, S. (2016). Physical activity patterns in the elderly Kashan population. *Iranian Red Crescent Medical Journal*, 18(6), e25008.

Salehi, L., Taghdisi, M. H., Ghasemi, H., & Shokervash, B. (2010). To identify the facilitator and barrier factors of physical activity among elderly people in Tehran. *Iranian Journal of Epidemiology*, 6(2), 7–15.

Scarborough, P., Bhatnagar, P., Wickramasinghe, K. K., Allender, S., Foster, C., & Rayner, M. (2011). The economic burden of ill health due to diet, physical inactivity, smoking, alcohol and obesity in the UK: an update to 2006–07 NHS costs. *Journal of Public Health*, 33(4), 527–535.

Schutzer, K. A. & Graves, B. S. (2004). Barriers and motivations to exercise in older adults. *Preventive Medicine*, 39(5), 1056–1061.

Seniors BC. (2012). Active aging—physical activity. Retrieved from: www.seniorsbc.ca/activeaging/physical/.

Sethi, D., Wood, S., Mitis, F., Bellis, M., Penhale, B., Marmolejo, I. I., & Kärki, F. U. (2011). European report on preventing elder maltreatment. *World Health Organization*.

Siddiqi, Z., Tiro, J. A., & Shuval, K. (2011). Understanding impediments and enablers to physical activity among African American adults: a systematic review of qualitative studies. *Health Education Research*, 26(6), 1010–1024.

Singh, M. A. F. (2002). Exercise comes of age rationale and recommendations for a geriatric exercise prescription. *The Journals of Gerontology Series A: Biological Sciences and Medical Sciences*, 57(5), M262–M282.

Skevington, S. M., Lotfy, M., & O'Connell, K. A. (2004). The World Health Organization's WHOQOL-BREF quality of life assessment: psychometric properties and results of the international field trial. A report from the WHOQOL group. *Quality of life Research*, *13*(2), 299–310.

Sohofi Parast, M. (2008). Iran pension system, current and future situation. In *International Conference on Insurance Industry*, 1–11. Retrieved from: https://slideblast.com/queue/iran-pension-system-current-and-future-situation_5975fad71723ddfe84277efd.html.

Song, Y., Ma, W., Yi, X., Wang, S., Sun, X., Tian, J., & Marley, G. (2013). Chronic diseases knowledge and related factors among the elderly in Jinan, China. *PLoS One*, *8*(6), e68599.

Spirduso, W. W. & Cronin, D. L. (2001). Exercise dose–response effects on quality of life and independent living in older adults. *Medicine & Science in Sports & Exercise*, *33*(Suppl. 6), S598–608.

Statistical Centre of Iran. (March 2017). The President's Office Deputy of Strategic Planning and Control. National population and housing Census 2016. Tehran: The Centre: Selected Findings.

Statistical Centre of Iran. Retrieved from: www.amar.org.ir/Default.aspx.

STATISTICS, U. B. O. L. (2012). Labor force statistics from the Current Population Survey. Retrieved from: www.bls.gov/cps/cps_htgm.htm#unemployed.

Struber J. (2004). Considering physical inactivity in relation to obesity. *International Journal of Allied Health Science and Practice*. *2*(1), 23–28.

Tajvar, M., Arab, A., & Montazeri, A. (2008). *Determinants of health-related quality of life in elderly in Tehran, Iran*. BMC Public Health, 8, 323–331.

Timiras, P. S. (Ed.). (2007). *Physiological basis of aging and geriatrics*. Boca Ratan, FL: CRC Press.

Trost, S. G., Owen, N., Bauman, A. E., Sallis, J. F., & Brown, W. (2002). Correlates of adults' participation in physical activity: review and update. *Medicine & Science in Sports & Exercise*, *34*(12), 1996–2001.

United Kingdom Department of Health. (2004). National service framework for older people. Department of Health. Retrieved from: www.dh.gov.uk/assetRoot/04/07/12/83/04071283.pdf.

United Nations Office on Aging. (2003). International Association of Gerontology. Research agenda on ageing for the 21st century. Retrieved from: www.valencia-forum.com/raa.html.

Vincent, K. R., Braith, R. W., Feldman, R. A., Kallas, H. E., & Lowenthal, D. T. (2002). Improved cardiorespiratory endurance following 6 months of resistance exercise in elderly men and women. *Archives of Internal Medicine*, *162*(6), 673–678.

Walker, A. (2002). A strategy for active aging. *International Social Security Review*, *55*(1), 121–139.

Watt, H. C., Carson, C., Lawlor, D. A., Patel, R., & Ebrahim, S. (2009). Influence of life course socioeconomic position on older women's health behaviours: findings from the British Women's Heart and Health Study. *American Journal of Public Health*, *99*(2), 320–327.

World Health Organization. (2002). *The world health report 2002: reducing risks, promoting healthy life*. Geneva: World Health Organization.

World Health Organization. (2003). *Key policy issues in long-term care*. Geneva: World Health Organization.

Part III

Chronic conditions and the impact of physical activity and exercise

Coping with chronic illness in the twenty-first century

The global diabetes crisis

Jasmin Tahmaseb McConatha and Elizabeth Raymond

Introduction

A global increase in life expectancy has resulted in a greater number of older adults who are living with one or more chronic illnesses. Approximately 92 percent of older adults over 65 suffer from at least one chronic condition (National Council on Aging (NCOA), 2015). The six most common chronic conditions in the United States are heart disease, stroke, cancer, type 2 diabetes, obesity, and arthritis. As of 2010, seven out of the ten leading causes of death were associated with chronic conditions (Centers for Disease Control and Prevention (CDC), 2016). Incidences of diabetes, in particular, are on the rise. In the United States in 2010, 26 million individuals were diagnosed with diabetes (Bernstein & Munoz, 2016). The number of people diagnosed with this debilitating illness is expected to double by 2030, resulting in 50 million people men and women (Bernstein & Munoz, 2016).

More than 18 million people with diabetes are undiagnosed and approximately 79 million Americans have pre-diabetes (Bernstein & Munoz, 2016). Pre-diabetes increases an individual's risk of developing other chronic conditions such as heart disease (NCOA, 2015). Of those who are struggling with diabetes, 90 to 95 percent have type 2 diabetes (National Institute on Aging (NIH), 2015). Clearly there is a diabetes health crisis.

Research regarding the personal, social, and community influences that motivate and provide adults with the confidence and education on properly managing their chronic illness diagnosis is crucial to the future promotion and prevention of all chronic conditions including diabetes. Many chronic conditions such as type 2 diabetes are influenced by lifestyle factors such as exercise and diet. Diabetes rates have increased around the world, however the United States is currently among the top three countries with an extremely high prevalence (Haltiwanger & Galindo, 2012). While there are programs and services to help people develop healthier lifestyles, become more active, and manage their illness, this epidemic illness is far from managed, especially among older adults.

Researchers have identified several factors that influence the successful management of chronic conditions, such as type 2 diabetes. While type 2 diabetes is a condition often managed by a healthy lifestyle, researchers suggest that it is also one of the most difficult chronic illnesses to manage (Samuel-Hodge et al., 2000). Coping and adjusting to any chronic condition is dependent on the interaction of a multitude of factors, including an individual's personality, sense of self-efficacy, how he or she understands the illness, available personal and social support, cultural values, norms, and resources (Ridder, Geenen, Kuijer, & Middendorp, 2008). Illness occurs and is managed in a social and cultural context. Investigators indicate that when faced with serious illness, people with greater personal, social, and environmental resources tend to adjust more positively. This chapter focuses on a discussion on the impact of personal and lifestyle factors on the management of chronic illnesses, exemplified with a case study on type 2 diabetes.

Personality and personal agency in managing diabetes

Personality factors such as motivation, control, and self-efficacy can help people maintain a more positive outlook and cope more effectively with their illness. For example, older adults diagnosed with type 2 diabetes, who feel a higher level of self-efficacy and a degree of control over their lives, are likely to be better able to make life style changes in diet and activity levels which can help with illness management. Technological competence such as skill in using the Internet for health-related information can also be seen as a form of social support and can impact the knowledge and confidence that an individual has regarding their chronic illness. Education and awareness about diabetes management can influence a person's understanding of illness, the type and quality of care they might receive, the kind of support systems they tap into and how effectively they manage to make changes needed to cope with their illness.

The need to understand the emotional, physical, and personal context of this illness is crucial for those diagnosed with diabetes (Cheng & Boey, 2000). The responsibility for making lifestyle changes needed to manage one's diabetes diagnosis depends on the motivation, resources, and physical and social support of the individual. Diabetes presents a challenge to life satisfaction; it can lead to feelings of helplessness, isolation, and loneliness.

Self-efficacy theory and illness management

Personal and environmental sources of support interact with personality factors such as motivation, self-efficacy, and a sense of control to serve as a buffering source in times of distress. These buffers help to minimize distress and increase the effectiveness of illness management. Self-efficacy, an important aspect of social cognitive theory, can be useful in understand the successful management of diabetes. Social cognitive theory (Bandura, 1999) focuses on the intersecting influences of personal and environmental factors when coping with and managing a chronic illness (Gallant, 2003). Bandura (1994) has argued that self-efficacy is one of the most powerful explanatory agents in human behavior. Self-efficacy expectations are described as beliefs in one's ability to successfully perform a given behavior. Self-efficacy is a trait that has been researched in relation to an individual's overall well-being, specifically with regard to disease management and coping strategies (Schwarzer, Bäßler, Kwiatek, Schröder, & Zhang, 1997). Self-efficacy beliefs have been found to help individuals begin and maintain exercise regimes. They help men and women struggling with diabetes feel that their efforts are likely to result in increased health and overall well-being.

Self-concepts of efficacy have an impact on choices, the amount of effort invested in treatment, how long to persevere, and whether tasks are approached with optimism, confidence, or hesitation. Self-efficacy can impact a patient's motivation and persistence in managing their illness by believing that change is possible, that it is within one's ability to make such change, and that changes will significantly impact one's illness and improve one's health.

Behaviors, such as healthy eating, consistent exercise practices, and self-monitoring blood glucose levels, can have a significant impact on the health and well-being of older adults with diabetes. When an individual is diagnosed with diabetes, they determine how much they are willing to change and adapt their lifestyle habits in order to maintain their chronic illness. Self-efficacy can play a crucial role in the patient's decision-making process while facing their diagnosis. They can either take action, by setting a goal to properly manage their diabetes, or the patient can make the choice to view their diagnosis in a negative manner by not prioritizing personal and lifestyle changes needed to manage their diabetes (Olsen & McAuley, 2015). People tend to consider the outcomes of situations and how well they will accomplish a set of goals, while motivating themselves to succeed.

Those who have a high sense of self-efficacy will envision successful outcomes for their chronic illness diagnosis. However, those who lack a high level of self-efficacy may have more negative views of their chronic illness diagnosis, which includes foreseeing failure for themselves and putting emphasis on the ways in which their chronic illness can get worse and not better (Bandura, 1994; Olsen & McAuley, 2015). When faced with chronic conditions in later life, a high sense of self-efficacy is necessary to remain focused on a successful outcome, for exercising regularly, and is helpful in staying positive and motivated to improve overall health.

Control theory and coping with chronic illness

A sense of control has been found to have a profound effect on health. Schulz and Heckhausen (1996) have formulated a theory of successful aging that focuses on the development and maintenance of a sense of control. A sense of control is associated with feelings of effectiveness and competence. Control is viewed as an important factor that influences well-being in later adulthood. A number of scholars have written about how control affects health and adjustment to illness (Ferguson & Goodwin, 2010; Krause, 1990; Rodin & Langer, 1977; Zuckerman, Knee, Kieffer, Rawsthorne, & Bruce, 1996).

The health belief model (Becker, 1974; Jones et al., 2015) illustrates how perceptions of health and illness affect how individuals cope with their illness and manage their well-being. This model incorporates subjective factors such as a sense of control, which is related to perceived susceptibility to illness, perceived seriousness of health concerns, and perceived benefits of certain actions such as treatments or preventative behaviors. A sense of control can influence subjective health by providing an individual with protective attributional processes while they are coping with their illness (Ferguson & Goodwin, 2010).

According to researchers (Chew, Shariff-Ghazali, & Fernandez, 2014; Ferguson & Goodwin, 2010), control is one of the most important factors that determines an individual's reaction to the social environment. The attempt to maintain a sense of control over one's life is an important challenge for people of all ages, but it becomes particularly important when one has to deal with a serious life-threatening illness. Several investigators have addressed perceptions of control and its effect on the lives of older adults (Chew, Shariff-Ghazali, & Fernandez, 2014; Ferguson & Goodwin, 2010).

Being faced with a chronic illness poses a significant threat to feelings of control. Seligman (1989) argues that people who feel a sense of helplessness show behavioral, motivational, cognitive, and emotional deficits. A sense of control, on the other hand, has been associated with positive health consequences (Nugent, Carson, Zammitt, Smith, & Wallston, 2015). Those who feel a sense of control over their lives have been shown to avoid self-denigrating attribution, manage their negative emotions more effectively, experience less unhappiness, dissatisfaction, isolation, anxiety, and depression (Ferguson & Goodwin, 2010).

Personal factors such as self-efficacy and control influence a patient's understanding of illness as well as capabilities and goals set for illness management. Those who have a high sense of self-efficacy are more likely to envision successful outcomes for their chronic illness diagnosis (Olsen & McAuley, 2015). When faced with a chronic illness diagnosis, personality factors impact the ways in which men and women cope. The amount of stress a person experiences, their depression and anxiety levels, and their willingness to positively motivate themselves can fluctuate depending on other factors such as feelings of depression and helplessness, activity levels, and satisfaction with social relationships.

Rumination

The tendency to ruminate about one's misfortune has been found to be associated with poorer adjustment to chronic illness. Rumination has been described as the degree to which people experience intrusive thoughts, feelings, and images of their illness (McCullough, Bellah, Kilpatrick, & Johnson, 2001). The greater the extent of rumination about the illness, the more likely they are to experience fear, anxiety, and distress. Rumination is defined as repetitive thoughts about one's distress (Brinker, 2013). Rumination not only leads to an increase of negative emotions but may also inhibit goal-directed activity.

Carstensen (1995) found that older adults are usually more able to regulate their emotional experiences than younger adults. In later life men and women appear to have gained an improved understanding of emotional contexts; consequently, they are able to interact more selectively with the social environment. During later adulthood, people can develop more emotionally rewarding lives by selectively disengaging from non-rewarding activities and experiences (Prakash, Hussain, & Schirda, 2015).

Exercise and other physical and social activity can help optimize positive emotional experiences and minimize negative and emotionally unrewarding experiences. Having to cope with a serious health concern means that one has to confront the medical establishment and pursue unpleasant, painful, and anxiety producing treatments (Prakash, Hussain, & Schirda, 2015; Tahmaseb McConatha, McConatha, Deaner, & Dermigny, 1995). Studies have found that those who stay active, both physically and socially, are better able to manage the distress associated with interactions with medical establishments.

Adaptive coping and chronic illness

Researchers suggest that practicing and maintaining adaptive coping mechanisms are crucial components in helping those diagnosed with a chronic illness (Cheng & Boey, 2000). Recent studies indicate emotional coping may be an effective coping strategy when dealing with an illness. Talking and thinking about one's illness results in less distress and anxiety and is a more effective coping strategy. Staying active also promotes a more positive approach coping (Cheng & Boey, 2000).

Positive approach coping, also known as task-oriented coping, is identified by using task or problem-centered coping strategies, for example patients diagnosed with a chronic illness would be categorized with positive approach coping if he or she views their diagnosis as manageable and determines a plan of action in which they will begin to make proper personal and lifestyle changes. In contrast, a patient who has a pessimistic outlook toward their chronic illness identifies with negative avoidance coping, also known as avoidance-oriented coping. For example, a patient using this coping mechanism might find his or her diagnosis as being an uncontrollable, irreversible illness.

Negativity has the potential to lead this individual to focus more energy on escaping the duties of managing their illness in attempt to suppress their feelings of anxiety and uncertainty about their future health and well-being (Cheng & Boey, 2000). Avoidance-oriented coping is closely related to the final strategy of coping, which is emotion-oriented coping. This form of coping is displayed when an individual incorporates the regulation of negative feelings that surface when they encounter a new life stressor, for example being diagnosed with a chronic illness (Burns, Deschênes, & Schmitz, 2016).

The extent to which a person spends time ruminating about illness is dependent on cultural values, belief systems, and the availability of support systems and resources. People who have a strong support system may be less likely to spend time ruminating about their illness.

Social and emotional support

Personality factors alone do not impact how a patient copes with chronic conditions. Several other interrelated factors also influence coping. One of the most researched of these is the support available to a person struggling to manage a chronic condition. Most researchers agree that during stressful times those who have a satisfying network of social and emotional support experience less distress. Satisfying social and emotional support is an essential component in establishing and influencing the quality of life throughout the life span. Relationships with family and friends, community groups, and economic resources help to develop and promote feelings of social integration and well-being (Gallant, Spitze, & Grove, 2010).

By meeting a person's instrumental, as well as emotional, needs, social support helps to protect people, to some extent, from the negative consequences of stressful life situations such as chronic illnesses. Research has found that one of the important benefits of adequate social support is the help provided in coping with adverse emotional and psychological effects of diagnoses (Cheng & Boey, 2000). Support also plays a role in motivation, which has been found to be a factor that can have an impact on an individual's self-management and self-care of diabetes (Lynch, Hernadez-Tejada, Strom, & Egede, 2012).

Hobfoll, Freedy, and Geller's (1990) social support resource theory focuses on a person's attempts to obtain and protect his or her personal and social resources. In times of stress, these resources are perceived as buffers because they help a person to feel more in control and they also help manage feelings of pain and anxiety. Social support, moreover, provides a person with a sense of interpersonal connectedness. It helps to promote a more positive and valued sense of self. In times of need, men and women can rely on people in their support networks for help or assistance. People may also rely on their friends and family for help and information on health-related issues. Overall, social support helps people cope with stressful and traumatic life events such as a serious illness and prevents loneliness and isolation (Cornwell & Waite, 2009).

Indeed, support groups may mediate the negative impact of a serious illness. Social support may slow down the negative effects of health resulting in more positive outcomes associated with illnesses. Social support includes satisfying relationships with family and friends as well as emotional, social, spiritual, and environmental resources. Research indicates that people with greater social and cultural resources are able to adjust more positively to difficult circumstances (Vassilev et al., 2013). These support resources, of course, cannot be tapped unless they are available. Contemporary cultural changes and the proliferation of computer technology, moreover, have provided new forms of social support.

Computer technology as a source of support

In technologically advanced societies, having access to and the ability to utilize technological support can influence the ways that patients cope with a chronic condition such as diabetes. Computer technology can provide information, social and emotional support, and increase feelings of self-efficacy and control. In recent years, computer technology has served a buffering function. In 2013, 59 percent of older adults, aged 65 and older, used the Internet and 77 percent described owning a cell phone (Smith, 2014). Given the availability of the latest medical research developments on the Internet, diabetes patients who have the skill and the means to make use of social media can use this as an additional important source of informational and social support.

Being able to gather information about prognosis and care can decrease feelings of helplessness and increase feelings of control (Tahmaseb McConatha, McConatha, Deaner, & Dermigny, 1995; Zrebiec, 2005). Access to computer technology can also provide social and emotional support in the form of support and discussion groups. Men and women struggling with diabetes can share their experiences with others who are coping with similar difficulties. This participation decreases potential feelings of isolation and loneliness. These groups allow users to feel connected with individuals who are experiencing similar life events and challenges.

Internet support groups act as a third space for older adults with diabetes to interact, share stories and advice, listen, and have an addition of a knowledgeable resource that provides them with tips, background literature, facts, and ways to properly live a healthy and balanced lifestyle needed to cope with their diabetes. In the United States alone, 25 million American have been reported to have participated in an online support group and have had positive experiences while interacting via these online social communities (Zrebiec, 2005).

The Internet contains a variety of different platforms that offer information regarding health-related questions, concerns, treatment, and support. The major Internet technology companies, such as Google and Yahoo, offer lists and postings that can bring users to a specific support group and/or discussion group that relates to the chronic illness they are living with (Zrebiec, 2005). The information regarding a specific chronic illness, such as diabetes, that is found through reliable Internet sources is not only beneficial to the patient but also to his or her secure social support systems. Studies have found that Internet discussion groups were a helpful, valuable, and convenient tool to both those diagnosed with diabetes and their close support systems (Zrebiec, 2005). This chapter addresses the ways in which participants make use of available social and technological sources of support and information.

Religion and spirituality as a source of support

A sense of spirituality influences well-being across the life span and serves as an important source of personal and community support for older adults struggling with a chronic condition (Bergan & Tahmaseb McConatha, 2000). For example, religious involvement has been identified with a more positive outlook toward the future. During times of stress, spirituality appears to reduce a person's anxiety. People who express strong religious faith and involvement also tend to report greater satisfaction with life (Lynch, Hernandez-Tejada, Strom, & Egede, 2012). Religious involvement, moreover, promotes a sense of belonging of a community, which serves to buffer stress during difficult times.

Age and ethnic differences seem to affect the extent of religious involvement. For example, studies indicate that older African American and Hispanic men and women report higher levels of religiosity than older European Americans (Lynch, Hernandez-Tejada, Strom, & Egede, 2012). In fact, religious participation has been shown to be one of the strongest predictors of psychological well-being among African Americans (Koenig, Larson, & Larson, 2001). Church attendance has also been related to longer life expectancy for both African Americans and European

Americans. The relationship between life expectancy and religiosity, however, was found to be greater for African Americans.

Loneliness, isolation, and chronic illness

Social isolation and loneliness are common among older adults, especially those who have been diagnosed with a chronic illness (Stankiewicz, 2015). Forty percent of older adults over 65 have reported experiencing feelings of loneliness at least some of the time (Hawkley & Cacioppo, 2010). Loneliness, which is a feeling of distress during a time when individuals feel as though their social needs are not being satisfied by the personal and emotional relationships they have with others, can impact an individual on personal, emotional, and cognitive levels (Hawkley & Cacioppo, 2010). A primary consequence of being diagnosed and living with a chronic illness is feelings of loneliness and isolation.

In the absence of adequate support systems, illness may increase social isolation. For instance, those who have an absence of social support and social connections account for experiencing more feelings of loneliness and are more prone to suffer increased rates of morbidity and mortality (Cornwell & Waite, 2009). The health risks that coincide with social isolation increase as an individual ages, particularly as they are more prone to experience stressful life events and transitions, as well as complications with their health and disabilities. Those who are more socially connected have a larger network of people that they can rely on for support and feelings of connectedness, which can be a factor that helps individuals cope with their chronic illness diagnosis and management (Cornwell & Waite, 2009).

As people live longer, there is a need to explore and conduct more studies in chronic illness management among the adult population. Type 2 diabetes has reached epidemic proportions in the United States, even around the globe, especially among older adults. There are not a sufficient number of studies addressing the struggle that older men and women experience in their attempts to manage diabetes. The success of coping with any chronic illness, specifically diabetes, is dependent on the intersecting influences of illness severity, co-morbid conditions, personality factors such as self-efficacy, a sense of control, the existence of satisfying support, and a sense of spirituality, and physical and social activity levels.

Conclusion

Illness management is shaped by cultural background. Racial and ethnic differences influence how illness is understood and managed. To fully understand illness management, researchers must take into account the racial and ethnic differences of patients. Maintaining a sense of well-being is a complex challenge for anyone. It becomes even more difficult in later adulthood when people must not only cope with multiple health concerns such as such as diabetes. Three in four Americans, aged 65 and older, suffer from multiple chronic conditions (CDC, 2016). Many suffer from multiple chronic conditions. A chronic condition such as diabetes results in a re-evaluation of self as well as relationships with others and the social environment in general. Diabetes and pre-diabetes patients must confront a new and very different set of social and cultural expectations; in short they are faced with a new reality with which they must come to terms.

Practitioners and program planners in the USA must take further steps to address illness management for older Americans. For many older adults, physical activity and exercise leads to increased psychological well-being, a higher sense of self-efficacy, greater motivation to make lifestyle changes, and an increased feeling of control. Staying physically active results in both primary and secondary prevention and health promotion. For those struggling with chronic conditions, studies have found that both morbidity and mortality are influenced by moderate regular exercise. In short, active living promotes a greater well-being and increased ability to cope with chronic later life conditions.

References

Bandura, A. (1994). Self-efficacy. In V. S. Ramachaudran (Ed.), *Encyclopedia of Human Behaviour*, 4, 71–81. New York: Academic Press.

Bandura, A. (1999). Social cognitive theory: An agentic perspective. *Asian Journal of Social Psychology*, 2, 21–41.

Becker, G. S. (1974). A theory of social interactions. *Journal of Political Economy*, 82(6), 1063–1093.

Bergen, A. & Tahmaseb McConatha, J. (2000) Religiosity and life satisfaction. *Activities, Adaptation, and Aging*, 24(3), 23–34.

Bernstein, M. & Munoz, N. (2016). *Nutrition for the older adult, 2nd ed.* Burlington, MA: Jones & Bartlett Learning.

Brinker, J. K. (2013). Rumination and reminiscence in older adults: Implications for clinical practice. *European Journal of Aging*, 10, 223–227.

Briscoe, V. J. (2014). Older adults and diabetes. *Diabetes Spectrum*, 27(1), 6–7.

Burns, R. J., Deschênes, S. S., & Schmitz, N. (2016). Association between coping strategies and mental health in individuals with type 2 diabetes: Prospective analysis. *Health Psychology*, 35(1), 78–86.

Carstensen, L. L. (1995). Evidence for a life-span theory of socioemotional selectivity. *Current Directions in Psychological Science*, 4(5), 151–156.

Centers for Disease Control and Prevention (CDC). (2016). Multiple chronic conditions. Retrieved from www.cdc.gov/chronicdisease/about/multiple-chronic.htm.

Cheng, T. Y. L. & Boey, K. W. (2000). Coping, social support, and depressive symptoms of older adults with type II diabetes mellitus. *Clinical Gerontologist*, 22(1), 15–30.

Chew, B., Shariff-Ghazali, S., & Fernandez, A. (2014). Psychological aspects of diabetes care: Effecting behavioural change in patients. *World Journal of Diabetes, 5*(6), 796–808.

Cornwell, E. Y. & Waite, L. J. (March, 2009). Social disconnectedness, perceived isolation, and health among older adults. *Journal of Health and Social Behaviour, 50*, 31–48.

Ferguson, S. J. & Goodwin, A. D. (2010). Optimism and well-being in older adults: The mediating role of social support and perceived control. *International Journal of Aging and Human Development, 71*(1), 43–68.

Gallant, M. P. (2003). The influence of social support on chronic illness self-management: A review and directions for research. *Health Education Behaviour, 30*(2), 170–195.

Gallant, M. P., Spitze, G., & Grove, J. G. (2010). Chronic illness self-care and the family lives of older adults: A synthetic review across four ethnic groups. *Journal of Cross Cultural Gerontology, 25*, 21–43.

Haltiwanger, E. P. & Galindo, D. (2012). Reduction of depressive symptoms in an elderly Mexican-American Female with type 2 diabetes mellitus: A single-subject study. *Occupation Therapy International, 20*(1), 35–44.

Hawkley, L. C. & Cacioppo, J. T. (2010). Loneliness matters: a theoretical and empirical review of consequences and mechanisms. *Annals of Behavioral Medicine, 40*(2), 218–227.

Hobfoll, S. E., Freedy, C. L., & Geller, P. (1990). Conservation of social resources: Social support resource theory. *Journal of Social and Personal Relationships, 7*, 465–478.

Jones, C. L., Jensen, J. D., Scherr, C. L., Brown, N. R., Christy, K., & Weaver, J. (2015). The health belief model as explanatory framework in communication research: Exploring parallel, serial, and moderated mediation. *Health Communication, 30*(6), 566–576.

Koenig, H. G., Larson, D. B., & Larson, S. S. (2001). Religion and coping with a serious medical illness. *Annual Pharmacotherapy, 35*(3), 352–359.

Krause, N. (1990). Stress measurement. *Stress and Health, 6*(3), 201–208.

Lynch, C. P., Hernandez-Tejada, M. A., Strom, J. L., & Egede, L. E. (2012). Association between spirituality and depression I adults with type 2 diabetes. *The Diabetes Educator, 38*(3), 427–435.

McCullough, M. E., Bellah, C. G., Kilpatrick, S. D., & Johnson, J. L. (2001). Vengefulness: Relationships with forgiveness, rumination, well-being, and the big five. *Personality and Social Psychology Bulletin, 27*(5), 601–610.

National Council on Aging (NCOA). (2015). Healthy aging fact sheet. Retrieved from www.ncoa.org/news/resources- for-reporters/get-the-facts/healthy-aging-facts/.

National Institute on Aging (NIH). (2015). Global health and aging: Living longer. Retrieved from www.nia.nih.gov/research/publication/global-health-and-aging/living-longer.

Nugent, L. E., Carson, M., Zammitt, N. N., Smith, G. D., & Wallston, K. A. (2015). Health value & perceived control over health: Behavioural constructs to support type 2 diabetes self-management in clinical practice. *Journal of Clinical Nursing, 24*, 2201–2210.

Olsen, E. & McAuley, E. (2015). Impact of a brief intervention on self-regulation, self-efficacy and physical activity in older adults with type 2 diabetes. *Journal of Behavioural Medicine, 38*, 886–898.

Prakash, R. S., Hussain, M. A., & Schirda, B. (2015). The role of emotion regulation and cognitive control in the association between mindfulness disposition and stress. *Psychology and Aging, 30*(1), 160–171.

Ridder, D., Geenen, R., Kuijer, R., & Middendorp, H. (2008). Psychological adjustment to chronic disease. *The Lancet, 372*, 246–255.

Rodin, J. & Langer, E. J. (1977). Long-term effects of a control-relevant intervention with the institutionalized aged. *Journal of Personality Social Psychology, 35*(12), 897–902.

Samuel-Hodge, C. D., Headen, S. W., Skelly, A. H., Ingram, A. F., Keyserling, T. C., & Jackson, Elasy, T. A. (2000). Influences on day-to-day self-management of type 2 diabetes among African American women. *Diabetes Care 23*(7), 928–933.

Schulz, R. & Heckhausen, J. (1996). A life span model of successful aging. *American Psychologist, 51*(7), 702–714.

Schwarzer, R. & Jerusalem, M. (1995). Generalized Self-Efficacy scale. In J. Weinman, S. Wright & M. Johnston, *Measures in health psychology: A user's portfolio. Causal and control beliefs* (pp. 35–37). Windsor, UK: NFER-NELSON.

Schwarzer, R., Bäßler, J., Kwiatek, P., Schröder, K., & Zhang, J. X. (1997). The assessment of optimistic self-beliefs: Comparison of the German, Spanish, and Chinese versions of the General Self-Efficacy Scale. *Applied Psychology: An International Review, 46*(1), 69–88.

Seligman, M. E. P., Abramson, L. Y., Semmel, A., & von Baeyer, C. (1979). Depressive attributional style. *Journal of Abnormal Psychology, 88*, 242–247.

Smith, A. (2014). Older adults and technology use. Retrieved from www.pewinter net.org/2014/04/03/older-adults-and-technology-use/.

Stankiewicz, G. (2015). Challenges in self-care in older adults with diabetes. *American Nursing and Midwifery Foundation, 22*(7), 33.

Tahmaseb McConatha, J. T., McConatha, D., Deaner, S. L., & Dermigny, R. (1995). A computer-based intervention for the education and therapy of institutionalized older adults. *Educational Gerontology, 21*(2), 129–138.

Vassilev, I., Rogers, A., Blickem, C., Brooks, H., Kapadia, D., Kennedy, A., Sanders, C., Kirk, S., & Reeves, D. (2013). Social networks, the "work" and work force of chronic illness self-management: A survey analysis of personal communities. *PLOS ONE, 8*(4), 1–13.

Wen, L. K., Shepherd, M. D., & Parchman, M. L. (2004). Family support, diet, and exercise among older Mexican Americans with type 2 diabetes. *The Diabetes Educator, 30*(6), 980–993.

Zrebiec, J. F. (2005). Internet communities: Do they improve coping with diabetes? *The Diabetes Educator, 31*(6), 825–836.

Zuckerman, M., Knee, C. R., Kieffer, S. C., Rawsthorne, L., & Bruce, L. M. (1996). Beliefs in realistic and unrealistic control: Assessment and implications. *Journal of Personality, 64*(2), 435–464.

Chapter 13

Education, physical activity, and healthy aging in Italy

Theoretical and operating dimensions

Antonia Cunti and Sergio Bellantonio

Introduction

The aging of the world population today is one of the most significant issues involving the whole social structure of the rich, industrialized, and technologically advanced countries. The drop in birth rates, as well as the rapid evolution of technology in the bio-medical field, has increased longevity, creating new development opportunities for the elderly and, therefore, unusual life expectancies. The increasing longevity of individuals, however, does not always lead to actual possibilities of social insertion, because of the popular ideals of efficiency and effectiveness on which the Western capitalist economies are based. From this perspective, longevity and aging represent two complementary factors that need to be adequately integrated: on the one hand, individuals now live for a longer time than in the past, on the other, they should grow old in the best way possible, in the belief that "health is a value in and of itself" (European Commission (EC), 2013, 1).

The aging experience is associated with the quality of the life that has been led and how well the individual has developed necessary skills that accompany a positive attitude toward age-related changes and transitions. Re-adaptation processes are continuing in adulthood and they are linked to biological changes and health conditions. Coping with new and unexpected life experiences requires a degree of self-transformation (Boulton-Lewis & Tam, 2011; Bowling, 2005). This chapter introduces the most advanced research perspectives in Italy that give aging as a phase of active adaptation and reconstruction. Furthermore, the way aging is experienced and managed by institutions in Italy is analyzed along with experiences and best practices.

As noted in neuroscience (Glees, 1968) and psycho-gerontology (Cesa-Bianchi & Cristini, 2014; Goldberg, 2005), aging involves not only processes of destruction and homologation, but also construction and differentiation: "One starts aging while growing up and continues growing while aging" (Cesa-Bianchi & Cristini, 2009, 14). Individuals get prepared for aging by developing skills related to resilience and by facing the continuous redefinition of human and social reality. Thus, "aging, understood as the systematic result of the interaction of biological, psychological, and social processes, is a lifelong process that begins at birth" (De Natale, 2001, 11). A positive image of aging as a process of self-realization, readaptation, and resource is far from the negative and stereotypical conception of aging considered as decay, and loss (Barret & Cantwell, 2007; Horton, Baker, & Deakin, 2007; Levy et al., 2002; Schaie, 1988; Umphrey & Robinson, 2007).

Creativity and aging

When attempting to understand well-being in later life the use of creativity is one important area of consideration (Cesa-Bianchi & Cristini, 2013; Cristini, 2012). Creativity involves multiple life domains including the ability to think differently about oneself, adapting to different contexts, coping with interpersonal relationships and the gratification that can be drawn from them. A key element in successful aging involves the motivation and ability to explore new opportunities of challenging the self (Havighurst 1953). Such an experience is always "individualized, conscious, and active" (Cesa-Bianchi & Cristini, 2013). Throughout life people need to overcome obstacles by acting on themselves and the surrounding environment. All existential transitions, moments of passage, the so-called "marker events" (Levinson, 1978), and the more or less radical transformations of our lives can take on different meanings and values—depending on the sense that an individual has given to life, or the way in which one has lived.

Aging does not constitute a univocal concept, to the point that it is difficult to answer the question of when it begins (Levi, 1998). It is possible to refer to the different changes that occur during the aging process. In fact, each stage of life can be interpreted from several points of view (Cesa-Bianchi & Cristini, 2014; De Beni, 2009; Laslett, 1992; Pinto Minerva, 1974, 2010). During the last decades, aging has become closely related to multiple issues of vitality (Scortegagna, 2005), such as liveability of senility, the possibility to know and be able to act until the end, to continue to grow and evolve, to use reason and fantasy, being interested in others and in the world, and to still be able to feel surprise and interest for life. Thus, aging is understood as an open and infinite evolutionary process. These positive aspects represent the potential for every individual; successful adaptation in later life depends on experiences and education, as well as psychological and social factors.

Everyone copes with later life in a different way, depending on the type of life lived during adulthood, the habits adopted during the lifespan (nutrition, physical activity, sedentary lifestyle, smoking, genetic heritage), but also on experiences, education, and culture related to the contexts of relationships, health, conception of self, and of an individual's creative, affective, and relational potential. Therefore, the transition from growth to involution occurs at different chronological ages for every individual. This justifies the concept of aging hetero-chronically (Cesa-Bianchi, 1998) being connected with the concepts of health and disease, and also to senility, including the most appropriate care practices.

Aging in Italy

In Italy, the stress associated with the current economic crisis has produced deteriorating living conditions for older adults. Studies have found that older Italians tend to be more lonely and poorer than in the past, mainly because of lack of resources. There is a need for institutions and local authorities to respond to the needs of older adults and to promote a better quality of life. This includes the dissemination of scientific research at the national and local levels, which is intended to implement best practices and verify social acceptance. (One such project is the *Perssilaa Project*, in which the Campania region and its university have cooperated.)

When it comes to aging, reference to the medical world and the way in which healthcare is managed is important. Although Western societies are clearly characterized by enormous progress in diagnostics and therapy, there is still an understanding of disease where the patient's role is limited to following clinical and drug prescriptions, while neglecting the fundamental role that every individual undertakes in relation to their state of wellness (Cunti, 2012).

People hardly see themselves as agents of their own health. One of the consequences of this mind-set of disease is that people are disengaged from their personal quality of life. And even after healing, people tend preserve the same life habits they had before the disease. Thus, the arrival of a new disease might be eminent and involves further appeal to physicians to adopt necessary therapies, often establishing a permanent vicious circle.

Health promotion needs to act on *empowerment*, understood as an individual's ability to exercise substantial power over personal wellness, which is also based on knowledge and awareness (Peterkin, 2012; Zannini, 2012). Hence, social responsibility is not insignificant; and the same can be said for healthcare systems, professionals, and for science dissemination. Although people have greater access and exposure to scientific information, the way it is presented often generates bewilderment and disbelief in the reliability of references. Health is, in fact, one of those areas where people have many different opinions and beliefs, which is specifically evident in discussion around nutrition.

As far as old age is concerned, it is often assumed that decision-making abilities are compromised and it is quite common to see the immediate family take on the burden of deciding about the health of its elders, who often refuse to follow the instructions/recommendations of their doctors and family. The most common attitude oscillates between a lack of confidence and distrust in the medical establishment, which is accused of lack of attention to individual cases and of following general protocols. Therefore, these patients eventually want to do everything by themselves, somehow. This situation confirms the need, not to pursue strategies of persuasion, but to enact strategies allowing individuals to be able to make choices, during the aging too (Demetrio, 2003). Moreover, it is well known that cognitive functions are better preserved if they have been used during our whole life; and the quality of knowledge learned through experiences will inevitably guide individuals' choices throughout the entire lifespan.

Importance of education

Currently, Italy experiences the need to combine the development of innovative therapies and diagnostics with general principles of well-being, such as nutrition, physical activity, and social life. This perspective represents an important educational value, with reference to the perception that people have of their own health. After all, they are the principle actors and have the responsibility of taking care of their own bodies and self. An education that focuses on the development of resilience will support elders in their ability to cope with and manage critical situations, and provide opportunity for personal growth. Such education should aim to combat what is known as "learned helplessness" (Seligman & Maier, 1976), namely the conviction that it is not possible to make any change. Unfortunately, this phenomenon of "learned helplessness" often leads to a permanent state of lamentation and complaints, and it is directly related to long waits in clinics, short doctor visits, costly medicines and therapies, incorrect treatments, inadequate health coverage, undesirable side effects of medicines and therapies, emotional coldness of doctor/health professionals' patient relationships, and early hospital discharges.

Hope

Another important factor to address in the educational process is the role that "expectation of life" (Dublin, Lotka, & Spiegelman, 1949) plays in the aging process. The hope for future life is a critical element conditioning the quality of the relationship between care-giver and patient; as it is no coincidence that the older the patients are, the more they complain about lack of self-care. In general, it appears paradoxical that older people who are retired from work do not dedicate enough time toward their own wellness. The time left to live is often characterized by a dilation of time, starting from the dismissal from work and often marked by a condition of isolation. Free time deriving from retirement and the end of other activities could serve as a resource, providing that one retains the ability and motivation to take care of oneself and to maintain important social relationships. As stated above, the quality of existence in old age is the result of what has been invested during the entire life.

These considerations reveal the urgency to intervene in the educational dimension of aging processes. In the health field, a vision of a truly educational problem is not always detectable. Generally, health professionals do not receive basic pedagogical training, as they are trained following a medical model that considers health as "the absence of disease" (Zannini, 2015). Thus, physicians and other health providers in Italy lack a psycho-pedagogical education, focusing mainly on the scientific, political, and regulatory side.

Bio-psycho-social model

According to a salute-genic model (Antonovsky, 1996), the health establishment and people are called into question for what they will do, especially in terms of the ability to balance the different parts of the Self. More specifically, the bio-psycho-social model (Engel, 1977) stresses the importance of psychological and social components, besides biological factors. Therefore, one must mainly consider the way in which individuals see themselves, trust themselves and others, and the gratification that can be drawn from their own existence (Lindstrom & Eriksson, 2005). In addition, an important indicator of healthy aging is the ability to restore forms of transitory balance, where the intellectual, emotional, and movement dimensions all interact with each other (Cunti, 2016). This allows for a "sense of coherence" in which all these components can be expressed. The the aging body needs to be accepted instead of views advancing "extreme youthfulness to the bitter end."

Healthy aging is a social goal. One of the guiding principles of the Ottawa Charter for Health Promotion (World Health Organization (WHO), 1986) is mutual support, understood as caring for others, territories, and natural environments. Health is a social investment as well as a community development; it is socially constructed through behaviors and human relations. All the systems within which individuals grow and interact are called into question, from the family, to educational institutions, and the work environments. Everyone is part of a social environment that conveys ideas and behaviors that influence the quality of life and, therefore, individual and collective health.

Wellness and welfare

Hence, it is important to combine wellness with welfare. Wellness, in fact, is a social issue because of how it can be promoted and how communities and societies equip themselves to satisfy the need and desire for wellness. Sport and physical activity, in particular, represent a powerful sensor of social and cultural change, and together they represent an emerging right of citizenship. In line with the Lisbon Treaty (WHO, 2009), this health model focuses on sports and physical activities, invoking a new model of citizenship. This wellness perspective focuses on community participation, innovative actions, and customized interventions, such as the introduction of physical activities and sports as an emerging right of citizenship. This means that sports should not be considered as a mere acquisition of techniques, but as a "social glue." Sports and physical activities are multifarious social environments (i.e., the values of sport and youth education, the creation of tracks in the environment to promote physical activities, and more). All these features are rapidly developing the consciousness to implement social policies that will encourage not only a better quality of life, but also a more equitable society, full of opportunities for the preservation of the environment and realization of the self.

Physical activity for aging in Italy—guidelines and best practices

Increasingly expressions such as *Healthy Aging*, *Happy Aging*, and *Active Aging* are becoming popular. Particlarly because of the scientific evidence on the topic of health promotion during an individual's lifetime (Bauman, Lewicka, & Schöppe, 2005; Paterson, Jones, & Rice, 2007), but also because of all the onsite projects promoting them. They indicate that strategies promoting healthy aging must be enacted through a bio-psycho-social intervention model (Engel, 1977). Engel's triplet, *Healthy-Happy-Active*, could be applied to the field of aging: where the word "healthy" refers to the proper maintenance of one's anatomical, physiological, and biological features; "happy" means to safeguard psychological well-being; and "active" refers to the promotion of an active lifestyle, including physical exercise and the pursuit of other healthy behaviors.

To discuss Italy's situation, it is necessary to first refer to the overall European framework, since it constitutes the frame in which our laws and territorial management work. Successful aging is particularly obtainable through movement and regular physical activity (Paterson & Warburton, 2010). For this reason, the European Regional Committee of the WHO has developed a more effective European Strategy for Health, highlighting some important information on "active aging," as a "leading European policy" on the issue of successful aging (Walker, 2009). Active aging was defined as "the process of optimizing opportunities for health, participation and security in order to enhance quality of life as people age" (WHO, 2002, 12). Thus, active aging

> applies to both individuals and population groups. It allows people to realize their potential for physical, social, and mental well-being throughout the life course and to participate in society according to their needs, desires, and capacities, while providing them with adequate protection, security and care when they require assistance.
>
> (WHO, 2002, 12)

Therefore, interest in an aging based on active wellness involves the elderly in the social, cultural, recreational, and physical activity fields, which help increase not only the state of well-being, but also the development of the entire population.

The importance of these issues has driven the European Commission (EC) to declare 2012 as the "European Year of Active Aging and Intergenerational Solidarity," with the intention of promoting an aging culture that values older people's contribution to society and to the European economy. "Awareness-raising and increased focus of political and public-policy agendas was underlined, as well as recognition and support to people already working on these topics, sharing of good practice, innovative approaches, and new synergies between existing players" (Tymovsky, 2015, 27). The European program particularly highlights public awareness about the issue of successfully aging. To do so, policy makers and stakeholders from Member Countries are urged to undertake, at all levels, actions to promote opportunities to improve aging and health.

Following the European guidelines, Italy has started several initiatives to improve the quality of life in aging, a goal increasingly urgent in the light of the very last demographic statistics in which Italy has recorded the highest share of elderly and very old people in Europe, second only behind Germany (Istituto Nazionale di Statistica (ISTAT), 2016). Many stakeholders expressed the usefulness of promoting "aging monitoring observers" to have an overall picture of the Italian situation and also to develop intervention strategies based on research as well as the latest guidelines issued by the EC (2013) and the WHO (2012).

In Italy, some importance was given to interventions in health education and healthy lifestyles through the collaboration among national health organizations, public research institutions, social welfare associations for the elderly, and those involved in the promotion and development of physical activities and sports. As for the observation and monitoring activities, "Passi d'argento" (Silver Steps) is a leading global monitoring unit of the status of health and disease of the Italian population over the age of 65 (Contoli et al., 2016). The project makes explicit reference to the WHO model on Healthy and Active Aging, which promotes the development of policy for the three pillars of active aging health, empowerment, and safety. The goal is to support an active view of aging and provide timely and scientifically valid data on the topic of prevention as well as indicators that measure the spread of prevention activities.

Monitoring involvement in physical activity

Italy's monitoring system describes the involvement in physical activity of people 65+ at the national and regional level through the Physical Activity Scale for Elderly (PASE). The questionnaire is divided into three sections: structured physical activity and recreation, social and household activities, and work activities (Logan et al., 2013). The most recent survey results (Contoli et al., 2016) confirm what had already been highlighted in the national and international scientific literature on the topic of physical inactivity (Physical Activity Guidelines Advisory Committee (PAGAC), 2008): health condition is related to numerous factors and their interaction, including traditional biological age, obesity, depression, and isolation—all associated with the decrease in the level of physical activity, as well as socio-economic and relational factors.

The data obtained made it possible to consider a set of useful factors to plan interventions in the field of physical activity for older people, to promote activities suited to this population. The instrument identified that Adapted Physical Activity (APA) programs are an essential strategy to educate the elderly in becoming more autonomous and enhancing existing capabilities (Winnick & Porretta, 2017). Such programs play an essential role in improving the life of the inactive elderly as well as of those suffering from chronic degenerative diseases, even after a rehabilitation cycle.

Adapted Physical Activity program

In Italy, the role and objectives of the APA program are indicated in the "Regional Guidelines for the Promotion of Health Through Physical Activity" issued by the Health Council of the Toscana region (2005) and declared as part of the integrated plans for public health. APA targets the population in stable health conditions. It is carried out in social communities in the form of group activities in places dedicated to social activities, including gyms, and requires the commitment of professionals in the field of physical education and physiotherapy. The recognition of such expertise has influenced the curriculum design in Exercise and Sport Sciences and has led to the establishment of several national projects regarding the quality of services provided by the Italian gyms, (such as "Palestra Sicura: Prevenzione e Benessere" (Safe Gym: Prevention & Wellness), promoted by the Region of Emilia Romagna in 2008). This service program highlighted the need to set up some so-called "ethical gyms," structures specifically engaged in physical activities and sports for APA program—under the supervision of appropriately trained graduates in Exercise and Sport Sciences. Because of the obvious and documented benefits of APA in successful aging (Winnick & Porretta, 2017), the Ministry of Health is trying to introduce these activities on the National Health Service level, as a means of promoting active aging. This can bring benefits such as reduction of the national health expenditure.

In line with this program, the University of Naples "Parthenope," in collaboration with the ARSAN (Agenzia Regionale Sanitaria della Campania/Regional Health Agency of Campania), the Universities of Foggia, Turin, Palermo, and "Foro Italico" in Rome, has started a counselling program for physical activity and APA projects. The focus is to introduce the APA program to patients with type-2 diabetes who are already monitored through the Percorso Diagnostico Terapeutico Assistenziale/Assistential Diagnostic and Therapeutic Paths (PDTA) program. Already after 1 year, the project results have shown significant benefits in the elderly people involved, as well as a reduction in the economic expenditures of the Regional Health Service, which include the decrease in the use of medication, medical visits, and prolonged hospitalizations (Liguori et al., 2014).

Furthermore, various associations in Italy are now concerned with the development of physical activities and sports, due to the organization by the Comitato Olimpico Nazionale Italiano/Italian National Olympic Committee (CONI). Several health promotion projects for the elderly have been created at a national and regional level, through an extensive distribution network of physical activities and recreational sports. The most important current projects are:

- *Luoghi di Sport* (Sports Places), which encourages the promotion of sports in the Italian regions with a limited number of sports associations and/or sport centers through physical activities and sports, including activities such as walking groups and APA programs;
- *Tavolo Nazionale di Promozione Sportiva* (National Board for the Promotion of Sports), which aims at the identification of guidelines on motor and sport activities, to facilitate changes of the entire Italian population's lifestyles; taking into consideration age, sex, and ethnic belonging in their planning, research, and training. This chapter aims to establish an organisational model based on multidisciplinary recreational and non-competitive activities.

(CONI, 2017)

Furthermore, the Unione Italiana Sport per Tutti/Italian Sport for All Union (USIP) promotes dissemination activities and paths of physical activity as an element of prevention and health promotion. For example, the

Area per la Grandetà (Area for the Elders) has started educational programs for active aging with psychomotor and cultural activities aiming at raising Italian elderly's awareness about new active and creative lifestyle. These programs are carried out in partnership with local authorities, municipal administrations, Azienda Sanitaria Locale/Local Healthcare Units (ASL), general practitioners, consortia, cooperatives, universities, and local associations. Practical activities include APA, senior fitness, home gyms, residential home gyms, walking groups, as well as groups against obesity and diabetic groups designed to educate older people about the importance of staying physically engaged and living a healthy lifestyle (Unione Italiana Sport per Tutti (UISP), 2017).

The following associations work together in Italy in order to achieve the goal of educating the elderly on healthy living:

- *Happy Aging* (Alleanza per l'invecchiamento attivo/Alliance for Active Aging) a member of the International Federation on Aging (IFA), supports intervention policies and strategies to promote and protect the health of the elderly, pledging to develop the indications for active aging. This alliance is designed as a cluster of organizations representing the bio-medical field and focusing on the wellness of the elderly, including Società Italiana di Igiene/Italian Society of Hygiene (SITI), Società Italiana di Geriatria e Gerontologia/Italian Society of Geriatrics and Gerontology (SIGG), and Società Italiana di Medicina Fisica e Riabilitativa/Italian Society of Physical Medicine and Rehabilitation (SIMFER).
- The following associations support healthy aging for trade unions: Federazione Nazionale Pensionati/National Retired Association (FNP), Confederazione Italiana Sindacati Lavoratori/Italian Confederation of Trade Unions Workers (CISL), Sindacato Pensionati Italiani/Italian Pensioners' Union (SPI), Confederazione Generale Italiana del Lavoro/ Italian General Confederation of Labour (CGIL), and the Unione Italiana del Lavoro Pensionati/Italian Labour Union of Pensioners (UILP).
- Associations focusing on the socio-institutional aspect of healthy aging include: Federazione Anziani e Pensionati/Elderly and Pensioners Federation (FAP), Associazione Cristiana Lavoratori Italiani/Christian Association of Italian Workers (ALCO), and Associazione Nazionale Comuni Italiani/National Association of Italian Municipalities (Federsanità ANCI).

All associations are working on the goal to improve and support a healthy aging process in the later part of life. This national *Happy Aging* project is based on five factors that promote successful aging: diet, physical activity, medications, immunizations, and screening (Happy Aging, 2017).

Conclusion

The testimonies presented here, albeit not representative of all the actions that are carried out on Italian territory, represent a significant cross-section of our country and are indicative of the fact that it is necessary to involve the political, health, social, education-training, and sports and physical education field to make a substantial change in a cultural direction. It is a major political and educational challenge to establish more cross-sectorial projects, as well as continuing with those that are already in place. The aim is to continue the reform of ideas that help better address the rapid economic, social, and cultural rights involving the elderly and promoting a "Community of Practice" (Wenger, 1998), through shared methods, research results, and intervention actions. Learning is not an individual process, disconnected from life contexts, but one that is based on *active* participation, and it is a constant reminder of concrete experiences. Therefore, a welfare system is needed at political and institutional levels that is able to regenerate the resources that are already available, empowering people who are receiving aid. This can increase the efficiency of interventions of social policies for the benefit of the entire community. One such proposal is "generative welfare" (Emanuela Zancan Foundation, 2016) that promotes the involvement of the person who is being taken care of as to contribute to generating resources.

This chapter highlights that investing in educational skills of the elderly and all those who are in contact with this population is of major importance to promote healthy lifestyles where the elderly are their own agents. The acquisition of these skills will have a generative value in the recipients later in life. Lifelong engagement in physical activities and sports can produce social values if they are not solely focused on performance but incorporate the aspects of care and guidance throughout the aging process.

References

Antonovsky, A. (1996). The salutogenic model as a theory to guide health promotion. *Health Promotion International*, 11, 11–18.

Barret, A.E. & Cantwell, L.E. (2007). Drawing on stereotypes: Using undergraduates' sketches of elders as a teaching tool. *Educational Gerontology*, 33, 327–348.

Bauman, A., Lewicka, M., & Schöppe, S. (2005). *The Health Benefits of Physical Activity in Developing Countries*. Geneva: World Health Organization.

Boulton-Lewis, G. & Tam, M. (Eds.) (2011). *Active Aging, Active Learning*. New York: Springer.

Bowling, A. (2005). *Aging Well: Quality of Life in Old Age*. Buckingham: Open University Press.

Cesa-Bianchi, M. (1998). *Giovani per sempre?* Bari: Laterza.

Cesa-Bianchi, M. & Cristini, C. (2009). *Vecchio Sarà Lei! Muoversi, Pensare, Comunicare*. Napoli: Guida.

Cesa-Bianchi, M. & Cristini C. (2013). L'anziano e le sue Potenzialità Creative. *Giornale della Accademia di Medicina di Torino*, CLXXVI, 317–330.

Cesa-Bianchi, M. & Cristini, C. (2014). *Come Invecchiare. Dalla Psicologia Generale alla Psicogerontologia*. Roma: Aracne.

CONI—Comitato Olimpico Nazionale Italiano (2017). Retrieved from www.coni.it/it/.

Contoli, B., Carrieri, P., Masocco, M., Penna, L., Perra, A., & PDA Study Group (2016). PASSI d'Argento (Silver Steps): The main features of the new nationwide surveillance system for the aging Italian population, Italy 2013–2014. *Annali dell'Istituto Superiore di Sanità. A Science Journal for Public Health*, 52, 536–542.

Cristini, C. (2012). Demenza e Creatività. *Ricerche di Psicologia*, 2–3, 563–576.

Cunti, A. (2012). Le Competenze Socio-Emotive nelle Professionalità della Cura. Una Ricerca Esplorativa relativa al Personale Infermieristico. *Educational Reflective Practices*, 1, 140–154.

Cunti, A. (2016). Mente, Corpo, Ambiente: Prospettive Pedagogiche per la Formazione di Corporeità Sistemiche. In A. Cunti (Ed.), *Sfide dei corpi. Identità Corporeità Educazione*. Milano: FrancoAngeli.

De Beni, R. (2009). *Psicologia dell'Invecchiamento*. Bologna: Il Mulino.

Demetrio, D. (2003). *Manuale di Educazione degli Adulti*. Roma-Bari: Laterza.

De Natale, M.L. (2011). *Educazione degli Adulti*. Brescia: La Scuola.

Dublin, L.I., Lotka, A.J., & Spiegelman, M. (1949). *Length of Life: A Study of the Life Table*. New York: Ronald Press.

EC—European Commission (2009). The Lisbon Treaty. In *Official Journal of The European Union*.

EC—European Commission (2013). *Investing in Health. Commission Staff Working Document. Social Investment Package*. Brussels. Retrieved from http://ec.europa.eu/health/strategy/policy/index_en.htm.

Emanuela Zancan Foundation (2016). *Cittadinanza Generativa. La Lotta alla Povertà – Rapporto 2015*. Bologna: Il Mulino.

Emilia Romagna (2008), *Palestra Sicura: Prevenzione e Benessere*. Retrieved from http://salute.regione.emilia-romagna.it/sanita-pubblica/piano-prevenzione/il-progetto-regionale-palestra-sicura.

Engel, G.L. (1977). The need for a new medical model. A challenge for biomedicine. *Science*, 196, 129–136.

Glees, P. (1968). *Das Menschliche Gehirn. Evolution, Bau und Arbeitsweise*. Stuttgart: Hippokrates.

Goldberg, E. (2005). *The Wisdom Paradox. How Your Mind Can Grow Stronger as Your Brain Grows Older*. New York: Simon & Schuster.

HappyAging—Alleanza per l'Invecchiamento Attivo (2017). Retrieved from www.happyaging.it/.

Havighurst, R.J. (1963). Successful aging. In R. William, C. Tibbits, & W. Donahue (Eds.), *Process of Aging*, New York: Antherton.

Horton, S., Baker, J., & Deakin, J.M. (2007). Stereotypes of aging: Their effects on the health of seniors in North American society. *Educational Gerontology*, 33, 1021–1035.

ISTAT—Istituto Nazionale di Statistica (2016). *Rapporto Annuale 2016. La Situazione del Paese*. Roma: ISTAT. Retrieved from www.istat.it/it/files/2016/05/Ra2016.pdf.

Laslett, P. (1992). *Una Nuova Mappa della Vita. L'emergere della Terza Età.* Bologna: Il Mulino.

Levi, A. (1998). *La vecchiaia può Attendere. Ovvero l'Arte di Restare Giovani.* Milano: Mondadori.

Levinson, D.J. (1978). *The Seasons of the Man's Life.* New York: Knopf.

Levy, B., Slade, M.D., Kunkel, S.R., & Kals, S.V. (2002). Longevity increased by positive self-perceptions of aging. *Journal of Personality and Social Psychology, 83,* 261–270.

Liguori G., Carraro E., Mammina C., Prato R., Romano Spica V., & Spinosa T. (2014). Counselling motorio ed Attività Fisica Adattata quali azioni educativo-formative per ridefinire il percorso terapeutico e migliorare la qualità di vita del paziente con diabete mellito tipo II. In G. Liguori (Ed.) *Il guadagno di Salute attraverso la promozione dell'Attività Fisica. Evidenze scientifiche e attività di campo-* Roma: Società Editrice Universo.

Lindstrom, B. & Eriksson, M. (2005). Salutogenesis. *Journal of Epidemiology and Community Health, 59,* 440–442.

Logan, S.L., Gottlieb, B.H., Maitland, S.B., Meegan, D., & Spriet, L.L. (2013). The Physical Activity Scale for the Elderly (PASE) questionnaire; Does it predict physical health? *International Journal Environmental Research and Public Health, 10,* 3967–3986.

PAGAC—Physical Activity Guidelines Advisory Committee (2008). *Physical Activity Guidelines Advisory Committee Report.* Washington: US Department of Health and Human Services.

Paterson, D.H., Jones, G.R., & Rice, C.L. (2007). Aging and physical activity: Evidence to develop exercise recommendations for older adults. *Canadian Journal of Public Health, 98,* 69–108.

Paterson, D.H. & Warburton, D.E. (2010). Physical activity and functional limitations in older adults: A systematic review related to Canada's physical activity guidelines. *International Journal of Behavioral Nutrition and Physical Activity, 11,* 7–38.

Peterkin, A. (2012). Practical strategies for practicing narrative-based medicine. *Canadian Family Physician, 58,* 63–64.

Pinto Minerva, F. (1974). *Educazione e Senescenza: Introduzione al Problema della Formazione alla Terza Età.* Roma: Bulzoni.

Pinto Minerva, F. (2010). La Vecchiaia tra Perdite e Nuove Possibilità Esistenziali. In L. Dozza & Frabboni F. (Eds.), *Pianeta Anziani. Immagini, Dimensioni e Condizioni Esistenziali,* Milano: FrancoAngeli.

Schaie, K.W (1988). Ageism in psychological research. *American Psychologist, 43,* 179–183.

Scortegagna, R. (2005). *Invecchiare.* Bologna: Il Mulino.

Seligman, M.E.P. & Maier, S.F., (1976). Learned helplessness: Theory and evidence. *Journal of Experimental Psychology: General, 105,* 3–46.

Tymovsky, J. (2015). *European Year for Active Aging and Solidarity between Generations (2012). In-Depth Analysis.* Brussels: EPRS. Retrieved from www.europarl.ie/resource/static/files/Events/eprs_ida-2015-536344_en-ep-report.pdf.

Umphrey, D. & Robinson, T. (2007). Negative stereotypes underlying other-person perceptions of the elderly. *Educational Gerontology, 33,* 309–326.

UISP—Unione Italiana Sport per Tutti (2017). Retrieved from www.uisp.it/nazionale/.

Walker, A. (2009). Commentary: The emergence and application of Active Aging in Europe. *Journal of Aging and Social Policy*, 1, 75–93.

Wenger, E. (1998). *Communities of Practice. Learning, Meaning and Identity*. Oxford: Oxford University Press.

WHO—World Health Organization (1986). Ottawa 1986. Report of an International Conference on Health Promotion. *Health Promotion: An International Journal*, 1, 405–460.

WHO—World Health Organization (2002). *Active Aging: A Policy Framework*. Geneva.

WHO—World Health Organization (2012). *WHO Handbook for Guideline Development. Geneva*.

Winnick, J.P. & Porretta, D.L. (2017). *Adapted Physical Education and Sport. 6th Edition*. Champaign, IL: Human Kinetics.

Zannini, L. (2012). L'educazione del Paziente. In A., Pellai (Ed.), *Educazione Sanitaria. Strategie Educative e Preventive per il Paziente e la Comunità*. Padova: Piccin Editore.

Zannini, L. (2015). *Fare Formazione nei Contesti di Prevenzione e Cura. Modelli, Strumenti, Narrazioni*. Lecce: PensaMultimedia.

Chapter 14

Achieving active and healthy aging in Sri Lanka

Malathie P. Dissanayake

Introduction

Development is a lifelong process of growth and change in physical, cognitive, emotional, social, and personality domains (Berk, 2010). Late adulthood, the last stage of human development, is both a time of growth and a time of loss. It is a time that many older adults feel they are able to focus on gaining emotional and spiritual satisfaction (Berk, 2007; Ryff, 1989). Unfortunately it is also a time of life filled with health challenges. This chapter will focus on the aging population in Sri Lanka, their health status, health and social challenges including changes in family structures, living arrangements, and the changing roles of elders in families and society. The promotion of active and healthy aging will be explored raising awareness of the challenges ahead.

Health status of aging population in Sri Lanka

As a country in the South Asian region, Sri Lanka has made significant strides in providing good health care to its population over the past decades. There has been a decline in mortality and an increase in life expectancy (Mittra & Kumar, 2004; Jayawardane & Bhuiya, 2012). The decline in mortality has been a result of various health programs including immunization campaigns, improvement in sanitary conditions, and eradication of malaria (Jayawardane & Bhuiya, 2012).

With respect to life expectancy, Sri Lanka has the highest life expectancy among the countries in the South Asian region (De Silva, 2008). Life expectancy as of 2011 for both men and women has increased markedly to 70.5 years for males and to 79.8 years for females, respectively (Ministry of Health, 2012). In many parts of the world, women have a higher life expectancy than men (Mittra & Kumar, 2004). Similarly, the majority of the elderly population in Sri Lanka are female (Abeykoon, 2000).

Increased life expectancy combined with a lower fertility rate has led to an increase in the older adult population of Sri Lanka. Considering the age structure of the population, the proportion of the elderly population (60 years and over) has significantly increased over the past few decades. In fact, Sri Lanka has the fastest-aging population among the countries in South Asia (Jayawardane & Bhuiya, 2012). It is expected that the older adult population will double from 1.7 million in 2001 to 3.6 by 2021 and the proportion of the elderly will increase from 9.2 percent of the total population in 2001 to 24.8 percent by the year 2041. Accordingly, by the end of the 2030s, one out of every four people in the country will be considered elderly (Jayawardane & Bhuiya, 2012). These changes have important implications, particularly when focusing on the health and well-being needs of older Sri Lankans.

Challenges of aging in Sri Lanka

Changes in family structure

Changes in the age structure of the country have also resulted in a number of changes to the traditional family structure in Sri Lanka. Previously older adults comprised a small segment of the population and were not perceived as "a burden." Those who needed care tended to be looked after by their families. Cultural values promote the family as responsible for taking care of its older members (Jayawardane & Bhuiya, 2012). However, this has changed over the past decades due to the increase of elderly population and the changes of family structure. Though there is an increase in longevity, the number of children in a family has also decreased. Hence, there are fewer family members to care for elders (Abeykoon, 2000). Consequently, it is challenging to provide adequate family support for older members, and this problem has been exacerbated due to migration and urbanization. The traditional family care system has also changed as a result of the increase in the number of women who work (De Silva, 2005).

These cultural transformations have resulted in the need for health professionals to find new ways to provide care for older adults in Sri Lanka. Focusing on self-care through awareness and education has helped. Providing necessary training and knowledge to groups (e.g., youth) who are able to look after elders, will help increase the quality of services for older adults living at home (Abeykoon, 2000).

Changes in the living environments—living with spouse and/or children

In Sri Lanka, the majority of older adults live with their children. According to World Bank Sri Lanka Aging Survey in 2007 (World Bank, 2008), 77 percent of older adults live either with spouse and children or only with children. About half of them prefer to live with their children and about

45 percent of them prefer to live either with their spouse or in alternative settings. Also, about 80 percent of all children think that their parents need to reside with them. However, there will be a decrease in co-residence of aging parents with adult children if level of education and income increase (World Bank, 2008).

Some older adults live with a spouse. It appears that these older adults tend to be better educated, more affluent, and younger. By the same token, older adults who are more educated, younger, healthier, and still employed also ones live with their spouse and children. By contrast, older men and women who live with their children appear to be older, less-educated, and widows. This group includes older adults with lower health status and those who have never been employed. Although older adults live with their partners and children when they are young, they also tend to live with their children later in life especially if they are female and widowed (World Bank, 2008).

A smaller proportion of elders in Sri Lanka live alone. Of those who do 75 percent are women. Most of these women are widows aver the age of 70. Also, most of them are retired or have never been employed and many do not receive satisfactory income. Studies have found that they generally tend to perceive their health status as either fair or poor. Two-thirds of them have at least one chronic disease or mobility problems (World Bank, 2008). Older women are at greater risk than older men. Similar to other Asian countries, a higher proportion of older women in Sri Lanka live alone, are less-educated, widowed, have lower income, and poorer health than older men. Older women in other Asian countries have poorer health status than older men (Bartlett & Wu, 2000). Therefore, they are more vulnerable than older men.

Changing role of elders within family and society

As a South Asian culture, respect and caring for older adults is considered an important cultural norm in Sri Lankan society. Thus, the respect and authority that they have in their family and in society are important aspects of their well-being. A key measure of the respect is their involvement in decision making within the family. According to the World Bank Aging Survey (2006) result (Siddhisena, 2005), two-thirds of elderly tend to discuss issues that are important within their families. Also, family members seek advice from elders on special occasions in the family (Siddhisena, 2005). Given the demographic transformation of Sri Lanka though, older adults feel that there is a decline in relation to the respect toward elderly not only in the family but also in society at large (World Bank, 2008).

Nevertheless, studies show that the majority of older Sri Lankans report being happy with the respect they receive from their families and friends.

It was reported that 92 percent of older adults think that they are important to their families and 80 percent of them think that they are important to their friends. Also, 80 percent of them have reported that they are satisfied with their family life. The satisfaction level of elderly in Sri Lanka is higher than other Asian countries. Family relations, social integration, and religious involvement may contribute to their high level of satisfaction. About 59 percent of Sri Lankan older adults feel that they are a leader of the family. If they are still employed, receive a pension, or own a house, they are more likely to become the head of the family, thereby influencing the decision making process (World Bank, 2008).

Inadequacy of emotional support

With respect to elders' perceptions of care, the majority (95 percent) thought that their children should look after them. Almost all older adults believe that they will receive emotional support when they are ill. However, a smaller proportion of older adults (13 percent) received emotional support as the main support from their families. For those who do not live with children, there is hesitation to contact their children when in need. As a result, these elders may not receive adequate emotional support from their families (World Bank, 2008). Emotional and relationship issues affect older adults' well-being (Perera, 2011). If these issues are left unanswered, they can lead to serious physical and psychological problems.

Most older men and women believe that they will be supported financially in case of need. They think that they will receive assistance from their children, partners, and son/daughter-in-law (World Bank, 2008). About half of older adults receive financial assistance, either non-pension government assistance or pension. Some depend on agricultural activities as their source of income. Those receiving pensions have a lower tendency to receive financial support from their children. However, older women have a higher propensity to receive financial support from children given that female life expectancy is higher than men and thus they may receive support from their children for a longer period. Older adults who are in need, disabled, in poor health, and those with a greater number of children tend to receive cash transfers and in-kind support (e.g., food, clothing) from their children (World Bank, 2008).

The majority of the Sri Lankan elders live in rural areas. Most of them work in the agricultural and non-formal sectors and, as a result, they may not receive a pension and other retirement benefits (Siddhisena, 2009). Consequently, they are more vulnerable in old age. It becomes the responsibility of the government to provide social protection for these at risk elders (Jayawardane & Bhuiya, 2012).

Support for daily functioning

Some Sri Lankan elders require assistance to carry out their activities of daily living (ADL) (e.g., eating, bathing) or instrumental activities of daily living (IADL) (e.g., cooking, traveling). About 44 percent are provided assistance to perform their instrumental activities (e.g., going to the doctor). Mostly, their spouses, children, and sons/daughters-in-law help them perform these activities. The support they receive tends to increase as they age. Older women receive more assistance for these activities. Grandchildren tend to support disabled grandparents, especially grandmothers. Older adults without children are provided support by their spouses, siblings, and other relatives (World Bank, 2008). Grandparents in turn also look after their grandchildren, an activity which keeps them physically and socially engaged. Studies have found that Sri Lankan older adults tend to look after their grandchildren similar to other Asian countries (Biddlecom, Chayovan, & Ofstedal, 2002). About 46 percent of older adults take care of their grandchildren. They like to support their grandchildren and consider it their duty. Also, they offer in-kind support (e.g., cooking, provide necessities) and financial support to their families (World Bank, 2008).

Health challenges of aging population in Sri Lanka

Older adults face various health challenges with age and, as a result, the country has the responsibility of providing care for them (Mittra & Kumar, 2004). Older men and women experience health problems such as hypertension, type 2 diabetes, cardiovascular and neurological diseases. They require healthcare including hospitalization, investigations, medical treatment, and post-hospital care and rehabilitation (Jayawardane & Bhuiya, 2012). Staying physically and socially active can promote health and well-being, and help older men and women stay independent for a longer period of time.

Prevalence of non-communicable diseases in Sri Lanka

Demographic transition in the Sri Lankan population has contributed to the change in the disease profile of the country. With the increase in the aging population, the prevalence of non-communicable diseases has increased (World Bank, 2008; Jayawardane & Bhuiya, 2012). Heart diseases, diabetes, and cancer are common conditions of later life (Mendis & Illesinghe, 1989; Balasuriya & Nugegoda, 1993; Nugegoda & Balasooriya, 1995). In 2001, 71 percent of all annual deaths in the country were due to non-communicable diseases. Conditions such as heart diseases, cancers, cerebrovascular conditions, and diabetes have been identified as main reasons for these deaths (Jayawardane & Bhuiya, 2012). Compared to developed countries, deaths due to heart disease are higher in Sri Lanka. There is a greater incidence of ischemic heart disease (IHD) among older adults compared to young persons (World Bank, 2008). Also, there is an increase in the prevalence of diabetes, particularly in urban areas in the country. It seems that one in five adults is has pre-diabetes or diabetes. Changes in lifestyle have considerably affected individuals in developing non-communicable diseases (Jayawardane & Bhuiya, 2012). Low levels of physical activity contribute to the high rate of these health concerns.

Considering the growth of the aging population, it seems that non-communicable diseases will increase in the future. Unless changes are made and older adults become more active and engage in preventative health care, these conditions will remain the leading causes of death (Jayawardane & Bhuiya, 2012). Chronic conditions also lead to an increase in frailty and disability. Older adults' frailty can have significant economic impact since it leads to physical dependence. It may increase the burden of healthcare cost as physically dependent elders require long-term care (Newman et al., 2006). Therefore, prevention of non-communicable diseases will result in reducing long-term healthcare costs (World Bank, 2008). Increasing activity levels, and providing information and education are important first steps in the process of managing and reducing the incidence of chronic illness among older Sri Lankans.

Elders' access to healthcare services

Sri Lankan older adults highly depend on public healthcare services compared to others. With respect to the healthcare visits of older adults, the World Bank Sri Lanka Aging Survey (2007) has revealed that 37 percent of visits were to a public hospital, 33 percent to public outpatient facilities, 23 percent to a private specialist and 11 percent to private hospital (World Bank, 2008). Accordingly, older adults, particularly those with a low income, highly use healthcare provided by government hospitals and other public sector services for their health concerns.

The use of healthcare services provided by the public sector seems to decrease with age. Lack of access to pensions and health insurance, lack of schooling, and unemployment may reduce the probability of using public sector services. Also, these services are not organized to offer continuous care for elderly patients. Thus, older adults may not have the access to a regular doctor. Further, they may not be able to do regular screening for diseases and disability since there is no system to coordinate and provide medical care for them (World Bank, 2008).

Sri Lankan adults seem to be more concerned about their health and tend to use healthcare services for their health problems (Dissanayake & Rupasinghe, 2016; Caldwell, Gajanayake, Caldwell, & Peiris, 1989). Although there is no regular system to screen older adults' health conditions, many elders diagnosed with chronic illnesses do relevant tests to ensure their health status. According to the Sri Lanka Aging Survey, 94 percent of elders with diabetes have tested blood sugar levels, and 93 percent of elderly with hypertension have tested blood in the previous 12 months (World Bank, 2008), suggesting high concerns and lack of motivation in health-related behaviors.

Disability and aging

Globally, disability is one of the main concerns among the elderly. The proportion of people with disabilities is rising as a consequence of population aging and chronic illnesses (World Health Organization, 2016). Chronic disease and disability are inevitable issues with aging. Researchers have suggested that the impact of disability can be minimized through successful interventions or programs such as improved medical care and treatment, improvement of educational level and socioeconomic status, positive behavioral modifications, an increase in exercise, and changes in diet, and use of assistive technology (National Institute of Health, 2010).

In Sri Lanka, the proportion of disability rises with the growth of the aging population (Abeykoon, 2000). The national population censuses conducted in 1981 and 2001 found that disability has increased among the older adult population (De Silva, Amarabandu, & Gunasekera, 2008; World Bank, 2008). In 1981, the disability rate was 99.1 per 10,000 and had increased to 199.1 per 10,000 in 2001. Both population aging and the civil conflict have contributed to the increase of disability. The history of chronic and other conditions also cause disability (e.g., blindness, and physical immobility) among the elderly; therefore, all efforts should be made for disability prevention and reduction (Newman et al., 2006; Abeykoon, 2000).

Aging is an influential factor that affects overall level of disability among Sri Lankans. As a result, the healthcare providers face various challenges since these changes have significant implications on addressing the needs of the elderly (De Silva, Amarabandu, & Gunasekera, 2008). There is a deficiency in resources and trained professionals in geriatric healthcare and an inadequate number of medical professionals. These challenges prevent improvement in the health status of older Sri Lankans (Jayawardane & Bhuiya, 2012). Disability among older adults in Sri Lanka is also gendered. The proportion of disability is higher in women than in men (De Silva, Amarabandu, & Gunasekera, 2008).

Blindness

Poor vision is a factor contributing to health concerns among older Sri Lankans. In fact, blindness is one of the most prevalent conditions among older adults in Sri Lanka (Mendis & Illesinghe, 1989; Balasuriya & Nuge-goda, 1993; Nugegoda & Balasooriya, 1995). Blindness among 50- to 69-year-olds has decreased from 1981 to 2001. In contrast, blindness among older aged adults (70 years and above) has significantly increased during this time period (World Bank, 2008). The censuses in 1981 and 2001 included individuals who were totally blind in both eyes. There was an increase especially for elders of 70 years and above, and a sharp increase was observed among those who are 75 years and over (De Silva, Amarabandu, & Gunasekera, 2008). Blindness is also associated with an increase in isolation and a more sedentary lifestyle.

Disability in hearing and speaking

Impaired hearing is another prevalent condition among Sri Lankan elders (Mendis & Illesinghe, 1989; Balasuriya & Nugegoda, 1993; Nugegoda & Balasooriya, 1995). Hearing impairment and speech disability among the aged have markedly increased from 1981 and 2001. Elderly who are speech and hearing impaired have also increased during the same period (World Bank, 2008). A noticeable increase was found from 17.4 per 10,000 people in 1981 to 55.7 per 10,000 people in 2001 among elderly. Disability in hearing and speaking has increased considerably from younger-old to older-old adults. With respect to gender, these disabilities were three times larger for older males in 2001 (19.1 per 10,000 in 1981 and 58.9 in 2001). There was a sharp increase in older females with these disabilities (from 15.5. in 1981 to 52.8 in 2001) (De Silva, Amarabandu, & Gunasekera, 2008).

It has been noted that noise pollution and occupational exposure can cause these disabilities among elders. During the last few decades, people in the North and East parts of the country were repeatedly exposed to intolerable noise associated with war, causing hearing impairment. Men tend to be more exposed to polluted environments than women; hence, the proportions of men with these disabilities are higher than women (De Silva, Amarabandu, & Gunasekera, 2008).

Motor disability

Other physical disabilities have been associated with poor health and lowered activity levels. These include disabilities of the hands and feet. Dis-ability in the hands comprises loss of one hand (below elbow), paralysis of one hand (complete inactivity of the hand), loss of both hands (below elbows), and paralysis of both hands (complete inactivity of both hands). Two types of this disability have been found among older Sri Lankans. One is the paralysis in one hand and the other is the paralysis in both hands. Hand disability has increased for men and women from 22.2 per

10,000 in 1981 to 48.8 per 10,000 in 2001. There was a sharp increase in this disability for elders of 65 years and over (De Silva, Amarabandu, & Gunasekera, 2008).

Disability in hands is on the rise among older women. There was a considerable increase for older women from 14.7 per 10,000 in 1981 to 37.1 per 10,000 in 2001. There was a greater increase in disability in hands in both sexes for elders of 65 years and over. Factors that caused an increase in this type of disability include civil war, bomb explosions, road accidents, factory and home accidents, and occupational trauma (De Silva, Amarabandu, & Gunasekera, 2008).

Disability in legs includes loss of one leg (below knee), loss of both legs (below knee), paralysis of one leg (complete inactivity of a leg), and paralysis of both legs (complete inactivity). The majority of disability in legs includes paralysis of either one leg or both legs. Recently, there is an increase in the number of amputations due to non-communicable diseases (e.g., diabetes). This type of disability has increased for both older men and women from 37.7 (in 1981) per 10,000 to 72.1 (in 2001) (De Silva, Amarabandu, & Gunasekera, 2008).

The increase in persons with non-communicable diseases may have contributed to the increase in disability among the elderly population. Disability in legs has increased among older women from 25.6 (in 1981) to 58.9 (in 2001) compared to older men. The increase was larger for elders (both men and women) of 65 years and above. The increase in the aging population may have influenced the increase disabilities in legs (De Silva, Amarabandu, & Gunasekera, 2008).

Promoting active and healthy aging

In Sri Lanka, free health services were introduced as a government policy in 1950 (Mittra & Kumar, 2004). The Ministry of Health together with the Provincial Council Departments of Health provides public healthcare services for citizens in the country. In recent years, the private sector has also provided services, mostly outpatient care, to the public (World Bank, 2008). The government had already taken several steps to face the problems associated with aging population. Offering well-organized, efficient, and systematic healthcare for elderly has an impact on reducing the economic burdens of providing healthcare and long-term care for elderly.

There is a greater need for an integrated management of primary care and prevention for older adults. It has been suggested that the primary care system needs to be utilized for the elderly, especially for geriatric assessment, chronic disease prevention, and other therapeutic interventions like rehabilitation. If the state provides healthcare services for the elderly with adequate and trained staff and necessary facilities it will help manage various aspects of chronic illnesses at the primary care level. In fact, if we are successful in managing chronic illnesses at the primary care level, it will be inexpensive compared to outpatient hospital care and inpatient care (World Bank, 2008).

It is also important to provide training for medical professionals, healthcare workers, and public health workers in elderly care in order to deal with these problems successfully. Geriatric care needs to be included in primary care and community care. Furthermore, Furthermore, a new primary care system based should be developed based on the utilization of well-trained family physicians in order to face new challenges of healthcare needs of elderly (World Bank, 2008).

The improvement of quality service in secondary care and prevention at public outpatient health facilities is also essential to improve diagnosis, necessary care, and treatment for poor and marginalized older adults. Disabled older adults and those among the old-old age may not be able to afford or access healthcare that is far from their homes. Compared to others, they need practical support to access these services. Therefore, if the state provides healthcare facilities which are easily accessible through public sector field officers, it will help minimize health complications as well as enhance medication adherence of elderly (World Bank, 2008).

Providing public financing for outpatient medicines and healthcare services, particularly for treatment of chronic diseases, is another important factor in reducing mortality and morbidity from these illnesses in future (World Bank, 2008). Expanding the health information system will also be beneficial to deliver information as well as evidence that are necessary to address the issues and needs of elderly population.

Developing policy for the elderly

Developing comprehensive and coherent policies is highly important in order to respond to the health challenges of aging. An organized system to address the needs of the elderly is a major requirement in achieving this goal. In 1998, the Ministry of Health appointed a director and gave specific responsibility to plan, implement, monitor, and coordinate healthcare services for elders. Strengthening the division for elderly care in the Ministry of Health is also important in this process. Accordingly, activities such as raising awareness of issues and challenges of aging to the government, medicines, availability of non-communicable diseases, and developing heath information systems and methods to link up with donors to address the issues of aging have been proposed and prioritized to meet the needs of elderly healthcare (World Bank, 2008).

The government has already taken steps to face the issues of an aging population. The Ministry of Social Services has initiated various programs covering three main areas: legislation to protect older adults' rights; establishing special secretariat for them; and initiating programs to support and improve living conditions of older adults. Enactment of the "Protection of the Rights of Elders Act" (2000) is a major step taken by the Ministry. Accordingly, a National Council for Elders, a National Secretariat for Elders, a National Fund for Elders, and a Maintenance Board for Elders were established to address the needs of the elderly. The legal foundation has been provided to develop a national policy for elderly in the country (Ministries of Social Services and Health, 2012). As amended in 2011, the Act provided more rights for older adults in Sri Lanka.

Long-term care system for the elderly

The need of assistance for the elderly will rise as a result of several reasons. With rising longevity, elders may require more support, both medical and social, from their community. The ability to perform daily living tasks decreases as they age and, sometimes, these activities may be hampered by chronic diseases or other causes. This results in a greater demand for long-term care for elders. This may cause higher levels of stress among family members who look after them. Hence, it is important to initiate an affordable long-term care system to fulfill elderly needs. It will help both elders and their children to lead less stressful lives (World Bank, 2008).

Homes for the elderly

As previously stated, the majority of Sri Lankan older adults consider that it is their children's duty to look after them in old age. Therefore, they are not interested in considering a retirement home or residential facility. The number of institutionalized older adults, however, has increased during past decades (Siddhisena, 2005). Changing values in society, lower fertility, children's employment, and living in separate homes after marriage are some of the reasons for institutionalization. Both the government and local non-government organizations support elders' homes. Studies have found that these homes often provide residential facilities for younger, more active, and better-abled elders (World Bank, 2008). Those who unable to live alone or in their neighborhood but do not require around-the-clock nursing care are often drawn to these places.

In general, Sri Lankan culture still encourages co-residence with elderly parents. It is, therefore, important to provide information and support for the family as well as the aging individual. Caregivers or families can be rewarded to motivate them and to continue their assistance to elders in the family. New methods can be introduced to support them to live with their families. The capacity of elders' homes can be increased for frail elders and those who require long-term and institutional care. Next, providing special assistance and services such as medical, financial, and psychosocial support, support for instrumental activities, and activities of daily living for older women living alone will help them to manage their lives in old age. Also, a social security system can be introduced to help them lead a healthy life in old age (World Bank, 2008).

Special services for the elderly: home-care service

There is a lack of facilities, especially for elders who have mobility problems and are unable to undertake daily living tasks. Special care or long-term 24-hour care needs to be provided for them. Few places are available with these facilities. They seem, however, to be more expensive (World Bank, 2008). Thus, it is important to find affordable alternatives for these older adults.

The National Secretariat has started a home-care service to support frail older adults. A 24-hour hotline has been offered for these adults so that they can receive the service of trained caregivers. In addition, the divisional secretaries and the Ministry of Health have trained caregivers to provide home-care service for these adults. They can receive the service while they are in their own family setting. It gives them an opportunity to continue their life with their families and to enhance overall well-being (Ministries of Social Services and Health, 2012).

Training for health professionals in elderly care

In Sri Lanka, like many other countries, the number of healthcare professionals in the healthcare system is not sufficient to cope with the demands of the aging population (Jayawardane & Bhuiya, 2012). There is a shortage of geriatricians and healthcare workers with special training in geriatric healthcare (Perera, 2011; Jayawardane & Bhuiya, 2012). Hence, training for healthcare professionals, healthcare workers, and public health workers in elderly care is important to address elders' needs and to resolve their problems successfully. The Postgraduate Institute of Medicine, with the support of the Ministry of Health, has already taken action to offer postgraduate programs related to elderly medicine. Care for aging adults has been introduced into the undergraduate medical curriculum to equip medical undergraduates with knowledge and understanding about issues of aging. The public health workers are also given basic training in elder care to achieve this goal (Ministries of Social Services and Health, 2012).

Physical and social engagement in later life

Studies have found the older adults are generally satisfied with their social relationships (Ryff & Keyes, 1995; Ryff, Keyes, & Hughes, 2004) and they tend to gain emotional satisfaction by strengthening their relationships. South Asian cultures (e.g., India and Sri Lanka) are considered as more collectivist cultures (Markus & Kitayama, 1991; Miller, 1994; Freeman 1998) and researchers have found that Sri Lankans place considerable emphasis on the quality of their relationships (Dissanayake, 2010). Accordingly, older adults in Sri Lanka tend to be socially active and engaged in social activities, not only with family but with other social groups as well.

When considering social integration of older adults, investigators (Marmot & Wilkinson, 2006; Perera, 2011) have found that half of the participants are members of various social groups such as senior citizen's clubs and village development societies. They tend to participate in religious organizations, death donation society, and poverty alleviation programs. Those who are more socially engaged also tend to be more physically active. Lower levels of social engagement have been found to adversely affect overall well-being and to contribute to morbidity in old age (Perera, 2011). Promoting community activities, including participation in religious events, recreational activities, and other health-related activities, also promotes functional fitness activities and helps elders to maintain a higher quality of life in old age. A variety of programs and facilities have been established. These promote physical and social activity among Sri Lankan elders.

Elders' committees

In 2003, the National Secretariat initiated a program to establish elders' societies at village, divisional, and district levels in order to empower older adults, to protect their rights, and enhance well-being. These societies help them enhance their social, cultural, and spiritual development. They organize free health clinics, religious activities, pilgrimages, and other cultural events so that they can spend time with their companions (Fernando, 1995; Marmot & Wilkinson, 2006). Also, these committees help different groups in their community through various programs such as offering financial support for self-employment and housing to poor elders (Ministries of Social Services and Health, 2012). Older adults gain greater satisfaction by engaging in these activities.

Day centers for older adults

In other countries, adult day centers are designed to provide a safe and supportive environment, care and companionship, and activity for elders during the day. These centers were either established under the guidance of village-level elders' committees and others were organized independently. The main purpose of these centers is to provide a facility for elders to spend the day with their companions, to engage in activity, and to socialize with same age groups (e.g., recreational, educational, and cultural programs). These centers are used for various health promotion programs (e.g., health awareness and health screening programs, free health clinics) (World Bank, 2008; Ministries of Social Services and Health, 2012).

Raising awareness on challenges of aging

It is important to distribute information on aging and related topics among the public and older adults. Various programs (e.g., island-wide awareness programs, distribution of leaflets, and handbooks on elders) have already been organized in order to raise awareness on the challenges of aging population among older adults as well as the community. Several publications including handbooks and magazines have been published. For example, the handbook on "elders," which includes information related to disease prevention, positive aspects of aging, information on how to lead a healthy and active life, and information on the various services available for older adults was published and printed in three main languages; Sinhala, Tamil, and English (Ministries of Social Services and Health, 2012).

Educational programs (e.g., pre-retirement seminars) have been organized for older adults, particularly those who are reaching their retirement age, to understand how to face this transition, to prepare them for old age, and to learn how to lead an active, fruitful, and healthy life. Both the National Secretariat and the Ministry of Health have organized these programs. Older men and women as well as various professionals, including medical doctors, psychologists, and sociologists, have contributed to these programs and it has been very successful for near-retirement individuals.

Psychosocial support is offered by trained counselors through the Ministry of Social Services. These counselors work under divisional secretariats and conduct various programs for individuals who require psychosocial support. They have extended the counseling service by starting counseling centers, training active listeners, and conducting awareness programs for various groups (e.g., teachers and public sector officers). More importantly, the National Secretariat has started a separate counseling unit to offer counseling for elders. A book on counseling for elders published in 2009 helps caregivers develop skills and gain better understanding of elders (Ministries of Social Services and Health, 2012). All these activities help elders to cope with daily hassles and to receive support and guidance to improve their well-being.

Conclusion

Sri Lanka has become one of the most rapidly aging countries in the world. This has posed new challenges including economic, social, cultural, and environmental changes that require special plans of actions to reduce the burden of an aging population. The rise in non-communicable diseases and disability resulting from the aging population in the country is one of the emerging health challenges that requires the most attention as well as resources. Identifying effective and sustainable strategies to fulfill the psychosocial needs of the elderly will be helpful for an active and healthy life. Good health care and social services, social security system, and opportunities and facilities for lifelong learning will help older adults to manage their lives, thereby experiencing optimal aging.

References

Abeykoon, A. T. P. L. (2000). Aging and the health sector in Sri Lanka: Meeting the challenges calls for fresh thinking and focused strategies. *Ceylon Medical Journal, 45*, 52–54.

Balasuriya S. & Nugegoda, D. B. (1993). Health aspects of an urban elderly population. *Ceylon Medical Journal, 38*, 29–30.

Bartlett, H. P. & Wu, S. (2000). Ageing and aged care in Taiwan. In D. R. Phillips (Ed.), *Aging in the Asia-Pacific region: Issues, policies and future trends*, (pp. 210–222). London: Routledge.

Berk, L. E. (2007). *Development through the lifespan* (4th Ed.). Boston, MA: Allyn & Bacon.

Berk, L. E. (2010). *Exploring lifespan development*. Boston, MA: Allyn & Bacon.

Biddlecom, A., Chayovan, N., & Ofstedal, M. B. (2002). Intergenerational support and transfers. In A. I. Hermalin (Ed.), *The well-being of the old persons in Asia*, (pp. 185–229). Ann Arbor, MI: University of Michigan Press.

Caldwell, J., Gajanayake, I., Caldwell, P., & Peiris, I. (1989). Sensitization to illness and the risk of death: An explanation for Sri Lanka's approach to good health for all. *Social Science and Medicine, 28*, 365–379.

De Silva, W. I. (2005). Family transition in South Asia: Provision of special services and social protection. *Asia-Pacific Population Journal, 20*, 13–16.

De Silva, W. I. (2008). *Construction and analysis of national and district life tables of Sri Lanka, 2000–2002*. Colombo: Ministry of Healthcare and Nutrition.

De Silva, W. I., Amarabandu, W.P., & Gunasekera, H.R. (2008). *Disability amongst the Elderly in Sri Lanka*. Sri Lanka: Institute for Health Policy.

Dissanayake, M. P. (2010). *Cross-cultural investigation of emotion differentiation and relationship quality*. (Unpublished doctoral dissertation). North Carolina State University, NC, USA.

Dissanayake, M. P. & Rupasinghe, P. D. (2016). The effect of health beliefs on self-efficacy and life satisfaction. *SAITM Medical Journal, 1*, 4–7.

Fernando, D. N. (1995). Support for the elderly in Sri Lanka. *World Health Forum, 16*, 1363.

Freeman, M. A. (1998). Linking self and social structure: A psychological perspective on social identity in Sri Lanka. *Journal of Cross-Cultural Psychology, 32*, 291–308.

Jayawardane, A. & Bhuiya, A. (2012). *Health security challenges in Sri Lanka and Bangladesh*. Washington, DC: The National Bureau of Asian Research.

Markus, H. R. & Kitayama, S. (1991). Culture and the self: Implications for cognition, emotion, and motivation. *Psychological Review, 98*, 224–253.

Marmot, M. & Wilkinson, L. (eds.). (2006). *Social determinants of health*. Oxford, UK: Oxford University Press.

Mendis, N. & Illesinghe, I. (1989). Health and social aspects of the Elderly. *Ceylon Medical Journal, 34*, 95–98.

Miller, J. G. (1994). Cultural diversity in the morality of caring: Individually-oriented versus duty-based interpersonal moral codes. *Cross Cultural Research, 28*, 3–39.

Ministries of Social Services and Health. (2012). Promoting ageing and health—the Sri Lankan experience. *Regional Health Forum, 16*, 47–54.

Ministry of Health, (2012). *Annual health bulletin 2012*. Columbo: Ministry of Health.

Mittra, S. & Kumar, B. (2004). *Encyclopaedia of women in South Asia: Sri Lanka* (Vol. 5). Delhi: Kalpaz Publications.

National Institutes of Health (2010). Fact sheet—Disability in older adults.

Newman, A. B., Kupelian, V., Visser, M., Simonsick, E. M., Goodpaster, B. H., Kritchevsky, S. B., Tylavsky, F. A., Rubin, S. M., & Harris, T. B. (2006). Strength, but not muscle mass, is associated with mortality in the health, aging and body composition study cohort. *Journal of Gerontology. Series A, Biological sciences and medical sciences, 61*, 72–77.

Nugegoda, D. B. & Balasooriya, S. (1995). Health and social status of an elderly urban population in Sri Lanka. *Social Science and Medicine, 40*, 437–442.

Perera, B. (2011). Social support and social security issues of elders in Sri Lanka. *Galle Medical Journal, 16*, 20–23.

Ryff, C. D. (1989). Happiness is everything or is it? Explorations on the meaning of psychological well-being. *Journal of Personality and Social Psychology, 57*, 1069–1081.

Ryff, C. D. & Keyes, C. L. M. (1995). The structure of psychological well-being revisited. *Journal of Personality and Social Psychology, 69*, 719–727.

Ryff, C. D., Keyes, C. L. M., & Hughes, D. L. (2004). Psychological well-being in MIDUS: Profiles of ethnic/racial diversity and life-course uniformity. In O. G. Brim, C. D. Ryff, & L. Diane (Eds.) *How healthy are we? A national study of well-being at midlife*, (pp. 398–422). Chicago, IL: University of Chicago Press.

Siddhisena, K. A. P. (2005). Socio-economic implications of ageing in Sri Lanka: An overview, Working Paper no. WP105, Oxford Institute of Ageing, University of Oxford, October 2005.

Siddhisena, K. A. P. (2009). Aging population in Sri Lanka and its policy implications, In B. Weerakoon (Ed.), *ICPD—"15 years on" Sri Lanka: A review of progress*, (pp. 57–65). Colombo: Family Planning Association of Sri Lanka.

World Bank (2008). *Sri Lanka addressing the needs of an aging population*. Washington, DC, USA: World Bank.

World Health Organization (2016). *Disability and health*. Retrieved from www.who.int/mediacentre/factsheets/fs352/en.

Conclusion

Karin Volkwein-Caplan and
Jasmin Tahmaseb McConatha

Introduction

Physical and social activity is nothing less than a fountain of health. Public and scholarly interest in the promotion of physical activity across the life span has increased. Theories of aging address the importance of ongoing physical activity throughout adulthood. While there are similarities in the challenges facing international advocates of health promotion, there are also a number of differences with regard to resources, education, awareness, research trends, and policy (Tahmaseb McConatha & Sullivan, 2014). The chapters in this book address some of these similarities and differences. The contributors have attempted to explore the psychological, social, economic, educational, and cultural challenges that older adults face. They also suggest how institutions and governments can find ways to help elders meet those challenges.

Scholars have long addressed the health and aging concerns for those over the age of 65. The 14 chapters in this collection present an overview of programs that focus on the health needs of an international array of elders. In so doing the chapters address a diverse set of topics–chronic illness management, social activity, pain management, combating morbidity and mortality, and promoting longevity

Public health and aging

The median age of the world's population is increasing. By 2050 the average life span is expected to extend by another 10 years (CDC, 2013). The treatment of chronic diseases, which affect older people disproportionately, will put increased demands on the health care systems. Beyond the anticipated increased health care costs, it is time to make appropriate plans for public health programs to support the elderly and help improve the quality of the aging process. The authors in Part III of the book put forward particularly strong claims about a future health care crisis. They argue that proper plans and programs need to be developed to ward off the burden of future health care. One way to confront this problem, as the contributors to this volume suggest, involves regular physical activity, which has been proven to enhance and prolong life. In fact, physical activity has become a new *medicine*.

In the most industrialized societies, the maximal human life expectancy has increased from 49 in 1900 to almost 80 in 2017. As the chapters in this book suggest, lifestyle and the environment play important roles in the aging process. They affect our genes as well. In recent years, scientists have linked the shortening of telomeres to cardio-vascular disease, obesity, diabetes, and many forms of cancer and osteoporosis (Csatari, 2017). Gene researchers believe that lengthening telomeres might prevent these chronic diseases (Masood, 2011; Tzanetakou et al., 2014). Taking steps to optimize healthy aging can help protect telomeres. Indeed, the chapters in the book demonstrate that being physically fit, happy, and socially engaged can protect telomeres and, in turn, extend one's longevity.

Promoting healthy aging and longevity at the individual, local, national, and international level

That regular physical activity contributes to healthy aging is an incontrovertible scientific fact. It is equally clear that communities and governments need to promote physical and social activity. Physical activity is a *human need* and a *human right* and should be an important component of governmental policy and program planning. In addition, the promotion of physical activity should also begin at a young age. Research has shown that those who become physically active at a young age are much more likely to stay engaged in physical activity throughout their entire life span (Volkwein-Caplan, 2014).

At the *individual level*, the authors have pointed out that regular physical activity reduces stress, promotes healthy sleeping patterns, reduces of inflammation, decreases the risk for diabetes and obesity, and keeps people socially engaged and mentally alert (John Hopkins Health Review, 2016). In general, engagement in moderately intense physical activities (walking three times a week for 30 minutes, gardening, riding a bike, playing with kids, walking the dog, carrying heavy groceries, practicing in yoga and meditation) leads to an improved quality of life.

At the *local and regional level*, programs designed to meet the needs of older people should be developed. These would provide safe places where older people feel comfortable. Several contributors to this book suggest that it is wise to have medical professionals involved in program planning and implementation. Even severely injured or extremely disabled individuals will benefit from involvement in a program that addresses their specific needs or situations.

And at the *national level*, there is a need for financial support that will be used to promote the well-being of elders. Studies have shown that if older people feel that they are still contributing to society, they live happier, longer, and healthier lives (CDC, 2013). Those elders who remain in the workforce after 65 are more alert and experience a much slower decline in cognitive-control and social skills—because they "engage in control-demanding activities, including physical and social interactions with substantial degrees of uncertainly and surprise" (Hommel & Kibele, 2016).

The World Health Organization and the United Nations have addressed global trends in aging. They have also assessed how aging impacts demographic and epidemiologic transitions and increases medical and social costs. These, of course, have profound implications for public health; "the world has experienced a gradual demographic transition from patterns of high fertility and high mortality rates to low fertility and delayed mortality" (CDC, 2013, 101–102). This trend means that improvement in adult health has expanded the population of elders. Accordingly, now is the time to invest in this ever-growing part of the population. In more industrially advanced countries, the health care costs for persons aged 65+ are about five times greater than the rest of the population. In addition to addressing the increasing costs, public health agencies need to include in their future planning the health promotion in older adults, the prevention of disability, and the maintenance of capacities—programs for the general enhancement of quality of life.

Ultimately, all of the contributors have identified physical activity as the key component in promotion health and well-being. Physical activity, they suggest, helps to prevent diseases in older adults; it enhances the process of healthy aging. Given current demographic trends, public health program planners will need to consider whether they meet the needs of the aging population. Such programs will need to offer our elders: (1) safe spaces for physical activity programs, and (2) educational outreach on the positive health benefits of physical activity. The longer people consume unhealthy foods and lead sedentary lives, the worse off they will be in the later part of life (Sabia et al., 2014), which, in turn, raises the costs for their short-term and long-term medical care. All of the contributors argue that well-funded educational programs as well as the creation of environments in which health-enhancing activities can take place is of utmost importance. These smart investments will reduce the future costs of long-term health care programs. In the future, all people, no matter their age, their ethnicity, their gender, or their degree of disability should have access to spaces where they can freely engage in health-promoting activities. Our future quality of life will depend upon such access and participation.

References

CDC (2013). Public health and aging – trends in aging – United States and world-wide. February 14, 52(6), 101–106. Retrieved from: www.cdc.gov/mmwr/preview/mmwrhtml/mm5206a2.htm.

Csatari, J. (2017). Health & wellness: slow down aging. *Scouting*, May/June, 34–36.

Hommel, B. & Kibele, A. (2016). Down with retirement: implications of embodied cognition for healthy aging. *Frontiers in Psychology*, August 9(7), Article 1184.

John Hopkins Health Review (2016). *The Cult of Busy*. Spring/Summer, 3(1), 18–37.

Masood, A.S. (2011). Telomeres, lifestyle, cancer, and aging. *Current Opinion in Clinical Nutrition and Metabolic Care*, 14(1), 28–34.

Oaklander, M. (2016). The new science of exercise. *Time Magazine*, 188(10–11), 54–60.

Sabia, S., Elbaz, A., Rouveau, N., Brunner, E.J., Kivimaki, M., & Singh-Manoux, A. (2014). Cumulative associations between midlife health behaviors and physical functioning in early old age: a 17-year prospective cohort study. *Journal of American Geriatric Society*, 62(10), 1860–1868.

Tahmaseb McConatha, J. & Sullivan, J. (2014). Health and Fitness in Older Minority Adults. In: Guletta, T.P. & Bloom, M. *The Encyclopedia of Primary Prevention and Health Promotion* (2nd ed.). Charlotte, NC: Baker and Taylor.

Tzanetakou, I.P., Nzietchueng, R., Perrea, D.N., & Benetos, A. (2014). Telomeres and their role in aging and longevity. *Current Vascular Pharmacology*, 12(5), 726–734.

Volkwein-Caplan, K. (2014). *Sport|Fitness|Culture*. Maidenhead, UK: Meyer & Meyer Sport.

Index

Page numbers in **bold** denote figures, those in *italics* denote tables.

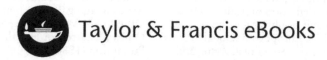

Milton Keynes UK
Ingram Content Group UK Ltd.
UKHW040103071024
449327UK00019B/766